DEPARTMENT OF HEALTH

ON THE STATE OF
THE PUBLIC HEALTH

THE ANNUAL REPORT OF
THE CHIEF MEDICAL OFFICER OF
THE DEPARTMENT OF HEALTH
FOR THE YEAR 1995

D0315386

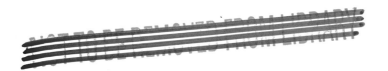

CONTENTS

INTRODUCTION

Rt Hon Stephen Dorrell MP
Secretary of State for Health

Sir,

I have pleasure in submitting my Report on the State of the Public Health for 1995, together with some comments on the more important developments and events in the first half of 1996. This Report is the 138th of the series which began in 1858.

I am pleased to report that health has continued to improve overall during the year. Infant mortality remains at the lowest recorded rate, and perinatal mortality and the rate of reported congenital anomalies both fell in 1995. Much progress continued to be made towards more integrated working to maintain the public health, and for more efficient communications between all those involved. The White Paper *The Health of the Nation: a strategy for health in England*[1] continues to provide an important impetus for improving health. Launched in July 1992, it has been taken up with vigour by a wide range of organisations. Encouraging progress has been made towards most of the targets set although, as is pointed out again in this Report, some targets present particular challenges.

As I have discussed in previous years, this Report is not simply a document of record, but must also try to interpret and to explain changes in those factors that are known to influence and to determine health, and should identify areas where improvements could be made. In recent Reports, I have highlighted some issues for special mention, with the intention that they would be followed up: topics identified in earlier years have been acted on and progress is discussed in this Report. As well as a broader discussion of understanding the language of risk, four other key issues are identified for particular attention during the coming year: mental health, antibiotic-resistant micro-organisms, information technology and HIV infection and AIDS. It is hoped that over the next year these four topics will stimulate interest, and I shall report back on these areas in next year's Report.

I wish to acknowledge the help and support given to me by numerous colleagues in the Department of Health and the Office for National Statistics in the preparation of this Report, and the assistance of Her Majesty's Stationery Office, Norwich, which arranged the printing and publication.

I am, Sir,
Your obedient servant

Sir Kenneth Calman

September 1996

1

LONG TERM STRATEGIC AIMS

Previous Reports[2,3,4] set out a series of long-term strategic aims which also underpin the content of this Report:

— To promote efforts to ensure health for all;

— To achieve the targets in the strategy for health;

— To involve patients and the public in choices and decision-making;

— To establish an effective intelligence and information system for public health and clinical practice;

— To ensure a health service based on an assessment of health needs, quality of care and effectiveness of outcome; *and*

— To provide a highly professional team of staff with strong education, research and ethical standards.

These six points continue to provide the strategic direction and intent of the Report.

HEALTH IN ENGLAND

Several key indicators of the overall health of the population indicate that the substantial health gains reported in recent years have been consolidated during 1995. The average expectation of life at birth was estimated in 1994 to be 74.5 years in males and 79.7 years in females; projections for 1995 indicate marginally lower figures than in 1994, but substantially higher than a decade earlier. The infant mortality rate reached its lowest ever level of 6.1 per 1,000 live births in 1994, and this level has been maintained in 1995 with post-neonatal deaths (deaths at 4 weeks to under one year-of-age) being at their lowest ever level. Perinatal mortality (stillbirths plus deaths under one week-of-age) also fell in 1995, to 8.8 per 1,000 live births and stillbirths, as did the rate of reported congenital anomalies - the provisional rate for live births now some 28% lower than in 1990, and that for stillbirths 10% lower than in 1990.

Nevertheless, there is undoubtedly scope for further improvement. For example international comparisons - as presented in Appendix Table A.11 - indicate longer average expectation of life in several other European Union countries, and lower infant mortality rates in a small number of countries (notably in Scandinavia). Consideration also needs to be given not only to the length of life but also to the number of years spent in good health[5].

A major theme that developed in the early part of 1996 was the identification, by the United Kingdom (UK) National Creutzfeldt-Jakob Disease (CJD) Surveillance Unit, of a novel variant of CJD[6]. Although CJD incidence figures for 1995 were, overall, well within expected limits, a new variant of CJD appears to have a younger median age at death, and the 10 cases first described had consistent clinical and neuropathological findings that distinguished them from other cases of sporadic CJD reported to the Unit. With one exception, the cases came to the attention of the Unit in the latter part of 1995 and in the early part of 1996; all had dates of onset of symptoms in 1994 or 1995.

The CJD Surveillance Unit was set up in 1990 by the Department of Health (DH) and the Scottish Office Home and Health Department, as recommended by the Southwood Working Party on bovine spongiform encephalopathy (BSE) in 1989[7], to monitor the incidence of CJD in the UK and in particular to look for any changes in the pattern of the disease in the wake of the BSE epidemic in cattle. It was vital that details of the findings of the new variant of CJD in the 10 cases first described were put into the public domain to allow them to be fully assessed by the scientific community both nationally and world wide. There was also considerable public interest. Much further work is required to understand the significance of this newly described variant. An important aspect of this is the co-ordination of surveillance activities both retrospectively and prospectively within the European Union (EU) and world wide, which is being actively pursued both by the European Commission and the World Health Organization (WHO). The UK has a key role to play, given its well-established and comprehensive surveillance system, and a programme of research on the human health aspects of transmissible spongiform encephalopathies, funded by DH and the Medical Research Council (MRC), is under way. It is important to ensure that initiatives in this area are fully linked with related animal health research programmes.

Regular statistics are now published by the Department to inform all clinicians of the findings of the CJD Surveillance Unit[8,9]. It remains impossible at this stage to predict the likely trends for reports of the new variant, or indeed for cases of CJD as a whole, and the identification of any aetiological factor involved remains a challenging but vital task. Measures to control bovine materials entering the human food chain remain a crucial element in the Government's strategy to protect public health.

THE STRATEGY FOR HEALTH

Since publication of the Report for 1994, a wide range of statistics have been released which enable assessment of further progress towards the Health of the Nation targets[1]. Of the 11 mortality targets monitored on the basis of routinely available data, eight have seen large falls in mortality since the Health of the Nation baseline (the average of the three years, 1989-1991). After allowing for changes to the Office for National Statistics (ONS) coding systems and procedures introduced in 1993, substantial reductions are estimated to have occurred for: coronary heart disease (CHD) in those aged under 65 years (19.2%) and among people aged 65-74 years (12.5%); stroke for 65-74-year-olds (14.3%); breast cancer in women aged 50-69 years (9.6%); lung cancer in men aged under 75 years (13.9%); suicide (7.7%); and accidents in those aged under 15 years (30.7%) and aged 15-24 years (25.2%). The other three mortality targets have also shown falls in mortality over the same period, but these will need to accelerate further to reach the targets. Stroke mortality in those aged under 65 years has fallen by an estimated 8.5%, lung cancer mortality in women aged under 75 years by 2.5%, and accident mortality in those aged over 65 years by 5.8% (although specific coding changes may make the last figure an underestimate).

Progress has also been good for many of the non-mortality Health of the Nation targets[1]. For example, conceptions among girls aged under 16 years fell by 5% in 1993 to the lowest recorded level for nearly 10 years; the prevalence of cigarette smoking in adults has continued to fall for both men and women (from 31% to 28% among men and from 28% to 25% for women between 1990 and 1994); and mean systolic blood pressure has fallen from 138 mm Hg in 1991-92 to 136 mm Hg in 1994. Particular problems, however, continue in relation to the obesity target - 1994 figures show 13% of men and 16% of women aged 16-64 years are classified as obese - and smoking prevalence among 11-15-year-olds increased to 12% in 1994, thus missing the 1994 target.

The fourth anniversary of the Health of the Nation White Paper[1] was marked on 8 July 1996 by a major conference with the theme 'Effective health promotion'. During the morning there was a meeting of the three major Health of the Nation Working Groups - the Wider Health Working Group (chaired by Baroness Cumberlege, Parliamentary Under Secretary of State for Health in the House of Lords), the Chief Executive's Working Group and the Chief Medical Officer's Working Group. As well as addresses from the chairmen there was opportunity for the Groups to mix and learn from each other about the different areas of activity involved in taking forward the strategy for health. The end of the morning was marked by the award of a prize to Mr Mark Weatherall from Cambridge, the medical student who won the national essay competition launched last October on the theme 'Health promotion in young people'. In the afternoon, the Lord President of the Council, who chairs the Cabinet sub-Committee on Health, announced the Government's intention to consult on a possible sixth key area on the environment in the health strategy. It is expected that this formal consultation process will start in October. Presentations were made on particular challenges, such as tackling obesity and teenage smoking.

In March 1996, bids were invited for an independent evaluation of the health strategy. A number of organisations indicated an interest to do work in this field and it is hoped that a contract will be awarded during 1996 with a view to publication of an independent review of the strategy for health in 1998.

In April 1996, the second Health Alliance Awards ceremony was held in London. Baroness Cumberlege awarded prizes to eight alliances and certificates of commendation to others. The ceremony helped to emphasise local enthusiasm and innovation for the strategy for health, and the use of local evaluation programmes.

In Spring, 1996, a briefing pack[10] was circulated to those working closely on the Health of the Nation intiative, with fact-sheets on the five key areas, an update on progress in these areas and descriptions of many of the different health alliances that are in place across the country. The briefing pack will be updated later this year as new monitoring data become available. A pack for general practitioners (GPs), produced at the request of the Royal College of General Practitioners and the General Medical Services Committee of the British Medical Association, was distributed to all GPs in March.

PROGRESS ON ACTION POINTS IN PREVIOUS REPORTS

Each year, topics which have been highlighted in previous Reports are reviewed and any action noted.

Progress on topics identified in 1992

The Health of the Nation fourth anniversary conference, described above, had *Men's health* as one of its three workshop themes. The Department will be considering the recommendations from these discussions; it has also arranged a conference 'Making gender matter', to be held later in 1996, to discuss and analyse the influence of gender in the purchasing and provision of health care and health promotion.

Cigarette smoking among men and women alike continues to fall, although the rate of decline shows signs of slowing. There are striking differences in prevalence of smoking between socio-economic groups: for example, 18% of professional men smoke compared with 39% of men in unskilled manual trades[11]. The Government's health promotion activity for adults, run by the Health Education Authority (HEA), is being increasingly targeted to reach groups whose smoking levels remain high. Smoking among 11-to-15-year-olds remains a particular cause for concern and a new three-year campaign was launched in 1996, which aims to use modern marketing techniques to question young people's perceptions of the attractiveness of smoking, and will be supported by initiatives with retailers to prevent illegal sales and by support for school anti-smoking programmes. New evidence continues to emerge about the health risks of smoking, and is kept under review by the Scientific Committee on Tobacco and Health, which reports to the Chief Medical Officer on the scientific and behavioural aspects of tobacco use, including the effects of environmental tobacco smoke.

Reports since 1991[12,13,14,15] have all drawn attention to the particular needs of *mentally disordered offenders* and the difficult problems they may pose to health, social care and criminal justice agencies. Such patients are only a small minority of the wider population of people with mental health problems discussed in this year's special chapter on mental health. In 1994/95, there were over 300,000 admissions to psychiatric hospitals, of which only some 2,100 or 0.7%[16] were via court disposals under the Mental Health Act 1983[17]. However, the severity of the disorder suffered by some can have a major impact on others, including patients, carers and victims, and can also profoundly influence public perception of people with mental health problems and of the mental health services[18,19].

Much has been achieved since the publication of the joint DH/Home Office report on mentally disordered offenders[20,21,22,23,24,25,26]. The number of medium-secure beds has increased rapidly from around 900 in 1992 to an expected 2,350 by the end of 1998. The number of patients transferred from prison to the National Health Service (NHS) more than doubled between 1990 and 1995, and the number of patients admitted as court disposals under the Mental Health Act 1983[17] increased by 25% over a similar period. Although co-operative working between health services and the criminal justice system has greatly improved, much remains to be done. There is also a need for a greater diversity of secure beds, particularly those offering longer term care at medium and low security levels. Mental health care in prison should be equivalent in quality to that within the NHS[27], and prison health care standards[28] have been set and must be met. The NHS and the Health Care Service for Prisoners are very closely linked by the need to ensure the availability of high-quality health care services to all offenders.

The Department has launched a research and surveillance programme in response to the Advisory Committee on the Microbiological Safety of Food's (ACMSF's) report on *verocytotoxin-producing Escherichia coli (VTEC)*[29]. There was a 93% increase in the incidence of VTEC serogroup O157 in 1995 compared with 1994; there is no obvious explanation for this increase, although improved ascertainment by clinical laboratories may have been a contributory factor.

Progress on topics identified in 1993

There has been increasing interest in the *health of adolescents* following the publication of the Report for 1993[30]. DH launched an initiative to target young people as part of the Health of the Nation strategy at a conference on 3 July 1995, and the Chief Medical Officer launched the 'Young peoples' health network' on 24 June 1996. The network is funded by DH and administered by the HEA. It will provide a forum for those interested in young peoples' health and, through the exchange of experience and ideas, should help to promote the health of young people and act as a catalyst for new work. A priority will be to ensure that young people themselves are involved and have an effective role in determining the network's direction and objectives.

DH continues to accord high priority to services for people with *asthma*. October 1995 saw the launch of a new NHS research and development strategy on asthma management.

Genetic factors and disease were raised to indicate their importance for health and health care. A number of developments have occurred (see page 215).

Changing patterns of infectious disease were raised in 1993 as a topic of particular importance and, in response to increasing concern about the international implications of changing patterns, and the emergence and re-emergence, of infectious diseases the World Health Organization (WHO) established a new Division to monitor and respond to new events and to strengthen national and international surveillance, foster research and co-ordinate responses.

Progress on topics identified in 1994

Health in the workplace: The special chapter in last year's Report[31] outlined some of the important effects of work on health, the effects of health on work, and the value of health promotion in the workplace. Risks from chemicals, radiation and other physical agents, and from biological factors, were outlined, and risk assessment and management highlighted. Continued progress by the Department and the Health and Safety Executive (HSE) is described on page 75; the importance of health and safety initiatives at work must still be emphasised to employees and employers alike.

Equity and equality: Last year's Report[32] raised the important issue of equity and equality, and set out a framework for considering such topics. The analysis was supported by a report[33] to the Chief Medical Officer on variations on health in England related to the five key areas in the Health of the Nation and the NHS. These made it clear that while inequity and inequalities exist, the evidence on appropriate interventions to improve such inequities is limited, and called for more effective local studies on how best to tackle the challenges. Equity, of course, has been at the heart of the NHS from the beginning. In its *Priorities and planning guidance* for 1996/1997[34], the topic is given particular prominence. In addition, the Research and Development Directorate has set aside specific funding to support research into variations in health status. There is considerable interest in the topic within the wider public health community, and in all parts of the country local projects are under way. Particularly relevant are the links which are being established between health and community development. Inner city areas, urban renewal projects, and rural initiatives show the value of partnerships and alliances in reducing variations in health. It is hoped that over the next few years such projects will bear fruit and indicate better ways to improve the health of the whole population.

Food poisoning figures remained stable in 1995 - the first time since 1992 that there has not been a marked upward trend. Field work for the major study of infectious intestinal disease in England has now been completed. Analysis of the epidemiological and microbiological data collected has begun and the Department should receive a report of the study, which will provide valuable information about the incidence and causes of food poisoning, in 1997. The ACMSF published its report on poultry meat[35] in January 1996. The report made recommendations, mainly addressed to industry, aimed at reducing the incidence of foodborne pathogens. An ACMSF Working Group has begun a review of foodborne viral infections and expects to report in 1997. The ACMSF has also begun to examine the implications for food safety of the increased incidence of antibiotic-resistant foodborne pathogens in human beings and food animals. The risk-based Food Safety (General Food Hygiene) Regulations[36] and Food Safety (Temperature Control) Regulations[37] came into force in September 1995, replacing 12 sets of regulations. The general regulations implement the EC general food hygiene Directive, emphasise the responsibility on food businesses to control risks, and set out essential principles of food hygiene (including the need for hazard analysis). The temperature control regulations introduced a single maximum chill storage requirement of 8°C, and replaced the list of foods requiring temperature control with a general requirement for food safety. The Regulations also contain flexibility allowing industry to vary temperatures under certain prescribed conditions which safeguard public health.

The DH tasks related to **_drug and solvent misuse_** arising from the three-year strategy for England, *Tackling drugs together*[38], are all on target and include the following initiatives. In the past year, 105 local drug action teams have been set up across England together with local community networks and drug reference groups; since late 1995, there has been an HEA national anti-drug publicity campaign particularly targeted at young people, and including the launch of a parents' guide to drugs and solvents[39]. The Task Force to Review Services for Drug Misusers report[40] was published in May 1996 and has been well received; its findings have assisted in the preparation of purchasing guidance for services for drug misusers. The 24-hour freephone National Drugs Helpline was opened in April 1995, and dealt with over 192,000 calls in its first year. Shared care arrangements for drug misusers between providers of primary and secondary health care have been reviewed by all health authorities, and medical and nursing professional bodies are helping to improve staff training and education. Deaths due to solvent misuse, which rose steeply from 1984 to 1990, fell again in 1994 when there were 57 deaths[41]; a further publicity campaign on the hazards of solvent misuse is due later this year.

NEW ISSUES IDENTIFIED DURING 1995

Each year a small number of issues will be identified as topics of particular importance, to be followed up in subsequent Reports. It should be recognised that the actions needed to ensure progress on these topics may be the responsibility of a wide range of organisations and individuals.

Understanding the language of risk

Most human activity is associated with risk - travelling, leisure, eating, working. Indeed some people enjoy risk, and deliberately take risks. How one describes and assesses these risks, what is meant by risk, and how one changes one's behaviour to meet these risks are important subjects. This section of the Report focuses on only one limited aspect - how to describe risk and the words used to compare risks, one with another. It does not attempt to review all aspects of risk, but does present a vocabulary for discussion and debate. This will be followed up over the next year and be developed further in next year's Report. But first some definitions. A hazard is a set of circumstances which may have harmful consequences. The probability of the hazard causing such effects is the risk of the adverse event occurring. A hazard is therefore a potential risk. The first set of issues to be considered, therefore, are those concerned with the assessment of risk; the identification of factors which might convert a hazard into a risk; the quantification of the magnitude of the risk to human health; and the need, if possible, to eliminate the risk. The result of this assessment is usually expressed as the probability of an adverse event occurring in the population at risk (eg, patients treated, individuals exposed). While this gives the probability of the risk occurring to an individual (eg, one in 1,000), it does not say whether this will, or will not, affect a particular person. A further issue is to consider the elimination of the risk. This part of the process is easily forgotten, but in some circumstances may be the most effective course of action. The third issue is that of the management and control of risk. This is generally done by the identification of particular points in the process which have been shown by experience to be of special concern - a hazard analysis critical control point (HACCP) process, which describes a very powerful method for the identification of critical parts in any procedure, or exposure to a hazard.

It should be clear however that despite such care, adverse effects can, and do, occur. Patients and the public should be aware that infections and environmental hazards, procedures, investigations or drug treatments do carry risks. Though the possibility of an adverse event occurring may be negligible (eg, less than one in a million), this does not mean that it might not occur to someone. This is generally not due to negligence or inappropriate treatment but to the risk inherent in the procedure itself. For example, not all clinical tests are completely reliable; false-positive and false-negative results do occur. The situation can, of course, be viewed the other way around. It may be, for example, that the chances of responding to a particular treatment are one in 20 or even one in 100. Even so it is possible, no matter how small the probability, that the treatment might be effective in the case of a particular individual. This may be welcomed for the patient concerned, but the implications for the population as a whole also need to be considered. For example, giving toxic treatment to 100 people with a particular disease in the knowledge that one may benefit has to be given careful consideration, in that 99 may be made worse in the process.

The most interesting but most difficult aspect of understanding risk is the perception of risk by the individual. Risks, no matter how clearly defined, can be interpreted differently by different individuals. Kant said "We see things not as they are, but as we are", and in doing so clearly described the problem. For example, the adverse health effects of cigarette smoking have been well described for four decades and are not contentious. According to most surveys carried out these facts are well known to the population as a whole, yet around 30% of the adult population still smoke. This contrasts directly with other health issues in which the actual risks may be very small, or of little general consequence, but the public radically alter their habits in response to a particular 'scare'.

There is also an important distinction to be made between relative and absolute risk, and this is perhaps best illustrated by an examination of the increased risk of venous thrombosis by combined oral contraceptives. It is true that the relative risk of venous thrombosis (defined as venous thrombotic episodes, VTEs) is doubled by the combined oral contraceptives containing desogestrel or gestodene compared with second-generation combined oral contraceptives. However, the absolute risk is very small in all types of oral contraceptives, and much smaller than the risk in pregnancy. The public presentation of these figures caused great anxiety; although the increased risk was small, women did need to be informed that there was a difference in risk betwen the oral contraceptives available to them[42,43] (see Introduction Table 1). The message, to continue to take the oral contraceptive pill, seemed to be ignored in the pressure for action.

Table I.1: *Risk of venous thromboembolism and mortality in women by contraceptive use and pregnancy*

	VTE per 100,000 women per year	Mortality per 1 million women per year
No OC use	5	0.5
Second-generation combined OC	15	1.5
Combined OC containing desogestrel or gestodene	30	3.0
Pregnancy	60	6.0

OC = oral contraceptive; VTE = venous thrombotic episode.

Source: Medicines Control Agency, from various studies

There is a further concern when the possibility of unknown or unpredicted side-effects is considered. These may happen many years after the treatment or exposure and may affect all or only a proportion of those treated or exposed. This is the nature of the development of new treatments or investigations. Their immediate benefit may be great and indeed may be demanded by the public, only later to realise that the long-term consequences may be associated with adverse events. Science is expected to deliver, but the public need to understand more about the nature of science, and the real differences of opinion which may occur during the often unstructured process of discovery.

The problem for decision-makers is not when the evidence is clear, but when it is weak or incomplete. In some instances no information at all is presented - only a hypothesis, or an idea which still requires to be tested, for example the suggestion that exposure to substance X may be related to condition Y, without any evidence being made available. In such instances of uncertainty two courses of action are possible: to go beyond the evidence and act in a precautionary manner, in which instance policy-makers act in advance of full information; or to wait until the evidence is clear before making this decision, a process which may take months or years. A particular decision will depend on judgment and will vary with the nature of the issue. In such instances there is a need for openness and sharing of information, and the establishment of trust between those who make policy and the public at large. This will sometimes mean that the fact that there is reasonable doubt, or that there is no answer to the question, may need to be clearly stated.

How then can risks be described and what does the language mean? Risks have been described in various ways - such as negligible, minimal, remote, very small, small and so on. Public and professionals alike are rightly confused by such a range of words. A classification is required to assist in the understanding of the process, but in so doing such terms need to be qualified by other words which may be equally important. These include:

— *Avoidable-unavoidable*: An important and clear distinction that can radically shift the perception of risk. Use of this dichotomy allows individuals to exercise choice, and for the public to be involved in the decision-making process.

— *Justifiable-unjustifiable*: These words implicitly carry values with them, and risks may be taken in some instances but not in others. For example, the use of a drug, with known side-effects, to treat a particular condition may be justifiable to achieve some benefit in some instances, but not in others.

— *Acceptable-unacceptable*: Once again these are value-laden words, but need to be used in a particular context. In general, an unacceptable risk would not be tolerated except for special reasons in special circumstances - for example, in the use of an unproven method of treatment as a therapy of last resort.

— *Serious-not serious*: Again these are words which refer to particular situations, but in this instance refer to risks which are life-threatening or likely to cause disability or morbidity, and those which are not.

Central to these concepts is the risk:benefit analysis and how this is perceived by individuals. Some individuals may not wish to take any risks in spite of the possibility of real benefit. Others will take a chance, even when the benefit is likely to be very low. With these provisos the following classification might be used. It draws on a great deal of other work, and is an attempt to answer the public's questions as to what is meant by safe. This classification is relevant only in relation to the description of risk, and not in relation to how that risk might be managed. It is put forward for debate and is not meant to be a final classification.

— *Negligible*: an adverse event occurring at a frequency below one per million. This would be of little concern for ordinary living if the issue was an environmental one, or the consequence of a health care intervention. It should be noted, however, that this does not mean that the event is not important - it almost certainly will be to the individual - nor that it is not possible to reduce the risk even further. Other words which can be used in this context are 'remote' or 'insignificant'. If the word 'safe' is to be used it must be seen to mean negligible, but should not imply no, or zero, risk.

—   *Minimal*: a risk of an adverse event occurring in the range of between one in a million and one in 100,000, and that the conduct of normal life is not generally affected as long as reasonable precautions are taken. The possibility of a risk is thus clearly noted and could be described as 'acceptable' or 'very small'. But what is acceptable to one individual may not be to another.

—   *Very low*: a risk of between one in 100,000 and one in 10,000, and thus begins to describe an event, or a consequence of a health care procedure, occurring more frequently.

—   *Low*: a risk of between one in 10,000 and one in 1,000. Once again this would fit into many clinical procedures and environmental hazards. Other words which might be used include 'reasonable', 'tolerable' and 'small'. Many risks fall into this very broad category.

—   *Moderate*: a risk of between one in 1,000 and one in 100. It would cover a wide range of procedures, treatments and environmental events.

—   *High*: fairly regular events that would occur at a rate greater than one in 100. They might also be described as 'frequent', 'significant' or 'serious'. It may be appropriate further to subdivide this category.

—   *Unknown*: when the level of risk is unknown or unquantifiable. This is not uncommon in the early stages of an environmental concern or the beginning of a newly recognised disease process (such as the beginning of the HIV epidemic).

Where precisely these terms fall in an individual case is a matter of discretion and debate. They may vary from time to time, with changing circumstances and information on the level of risk. It is possible, for example, for new research and knowledge to change the level of risk, reducing or increasing it. The use of these terms is further described in Introduction Table 2 which uses these terms to describe a range of different risks - some familiar, some less so.

The foregoing discussion leads naturally to a consideration of how best to communicate the level of risk associated with a particular health or health care issue to the public. The media have a very important responsibility in this regard. A number of guidelines have been described and they include: the importance of credible sources of advice, openness, sharing uncertainty, the need to accept the public as partners, careful planning, listening to concerns, co-ordinating with other credible sources and the importance of meeting the needs of the media.

It is hoped that this preliminary classification of the terminology relating to risk is of value, and that it will be the subject of further debate. However, it does emphasise the importance of ensuring that the public are full partners in the process of risk assessment and management, and it is only with such involvement that progress can be made.

Table I.2: *Risk of an individual dying (D) in any one year or developing an adverse response (A)*

Term used	Risk estimate	Example	
High	Greater than 1:100	A. Transmission to susceptible household contacts of measles and chickenpox[5]	1:1-1:2
		A. Transmission of HIV from mother to child (Europe)[2]	1:6
		A. Gastro-intestinal effects of antibiotics[4]	1:10-1:20
Moderate	Between 1:100-1:1000	D. Smoking 10 cigarettes per day[1]	1:200
		D. All natural causes, age 40 years[1]	1:850
Low	Between 1:1000-1:10000	D. All kinds of violence and poisoning[1]	1:3300
		D. Influenza[3]	1:5000
		D. Accident on road[1]	1:8000
Very low	Between 1:10000-1:100000	D. Leukaemia[1]	1:12000
		D. Playing soccer[1]	1:25000
		D. Accident at home[1]	1:26000
		D. Accident at work[1]	1:43000
		D. Homicide[1]	1:100000
Minimal	Between 1:100000-1:1000000	D. Accident on railway[1]	1:500000
		A. Vaccination-associated polio[3]	1:1000000
Negligible	Less than 1:1000000	D. Hit by lightning[1]	1:10000000
		D. Release of radiation by nuclear power station[1]	1:10000000

[1] The BMA guide to living with risk. Penguin Books, 1990.
[2] Peckham C, Gibb D. *N Engl J Med* 1995; **333**: 298-302.
[3] Immunisation against infectious disease. HMSO, 1992.
[4] Ness et al. *J Chemotherapy* 1993; **5**: 67-93.
[5] Harrison's Principles of Internal Medicine, 9th edn. 1975; 793.

Mental health

Mental health is an issue of considerable public interest. Various concerns focus around the care of patients and the public's understanding of the problems of those with mental illness, and of their carers. The incidence of mental illness and the range of services available are also topics of interest, and for these reasons the subject was chosen to be the special chapter in this year's Report.

A recent World Development Report[44] makes clear that across the world, even in developing countries, mental disorders (excluding drug and alcohol misuse) are a leading cause of lost disability-adjusted life-years, exceeding malignancy and cardiovascular disease, and accounting for 10.5% of all such lost years in males and 8.3% in females. The public health burden of mental illness in England, as elsewhere in the world, is considerable. Effective interventions exist which can reduce this burden, and it is therefore essential that mental health programmes and services are addressed and improved. The past year has seen progress on several fronts.

The Health of the Nation mental illness key[1,45] area has emphasised the importance of mental illness, and progress towards improving information and understanding about mental illness, developing comprehensive services and improving good clinical practice is being seen. The National Psychiatric Morbidity Survey is now complete (see page 96)[46], and the Health of the Nation outcome scale (HoNOS)[47,48] has been developed and is now available for assessment of progress in individual patients in a manner which can be used for more general assessments of progress towards the Health of the Nation target to improve health and social functioning of people with mental illness. A reduction of 7.7% in the national suicide target is most encouraging, although further progress needs to be made.

Mental illness is in the NHS *Priorities and planning guidance*[34], and purchasers of health care should ensure that the core elements of a local comprehensive service are in place in every health district. This message was reinforced by the Secretary of State for Health on 20 February 1996, when the Department published *The spectrum of care*[49] and a document about 24-hour nursed beds[50]. Implementation of the care programme approach and the Supervision Register, the continuing development of clinical guidelines for both primary and secondary care, and continued research into the extent, causes and treatment of mental illness will provide a sound basis for future progress.

Antibiotic-resistant micro-organisms

Methicillin was first introduced in 1959 and helped to curtail large hospital outbreaks observed in the preceding decade that were caused by penicillin-resistant *Staphylococcus aureus*. Although methicillin-resistant *Staphylococcus aureus* (MRSA) first appeared only a year later, MRSA strains remain only a small proportion of all *Staph. aureus* in the UK. In some other countries, particularly where antibiotics are more lavishly used, MRSA now comprise nearly 50% of all *Staph. aureus* isolations[51]. By the early 1980s, MRSA showing multiple antibiotic resistance and an enhanced ability to spread within and between hospitals were emerging and 16 of these 'epidemic' strains (EMRSA) have now been identified in the UK. Strains 1 and 3 caused large outbreaks in the mid 1980s, although each affected only one or two NHS Regions. Subsequent strains caused fewer problems and the number of isolates fell again by 1989. Strain 1 has now virtually disappeared, while the number of isolates of strain 3 has fallen to low levels. However, those designated EMRSA 15 and 16, first isolated in 1991-92, have spread widely and the total number of isolates submitted to the Central Public Health Laboratory has now risen above 1985-86 levels.

At least 80% of people who acquire *Staph. aureus* merely become colonised, not infected. About one-third of the population may be colonised with the organism in the nose or on the skin[52]; infection is no more likely to develop if the organism is an MRSA, rather than a methicillin-sensitive strain; and most infections are relatively trivial. The organism is not, therefore, a significant hazard for healthy people. However, hospital inpatients who are susceptible to deep infection, particularly if they have a surgical wound or catheters or devices penetrating the skin, may develop more serious infections, including pneumonia and septicaemia. MRSA infection can be difficult (though not impossible) to treat, and this difficulty justifies efforts to prevent such vulnerable patients coming into contact with it. Nevertheless, a recently published national prevalence survey of hospital-acquired infection shows no evidence of any overall increase since 1980 in infection rates as a result of the spread of MRSA[53].

Central Public Health Laboratory data show an increasing number of hospitals with incidents (defined as three or more patients colonised or infected with the same strain in a month) due to the commonest strains of MRSA. Not all incidents involve any cases of infection: nevertheless, hospitals need to take steps to prevent spread to at-risk patients and the risk of infection may require temporary closure of wards to new admissions. In some parts of the country, especially London and the West Midlands, adoption of strategies to achieve the necessary isolation of appreciable numbers of affected patients whilst minimising disruption to a hospital's normal routine has become a challenge, and providers of health and social care in the community have also become concerned that MRSA may be a hazard to their patients, which may lead to delay in discharging affected patients from hospital.

DH supports the clinical guidelines on the control of MRSA in hospitals published in 1990[54], and it formally commended these guidelines to the NHS in 1994[55]. It is now working with professional groups to revise the guidance to take account of the needs of hospitals with high and low prevalence of MRSA and of units with various degrees of risk. In May 1996, DH issued new guidance to providers of care in the community, recommending that people colonised or infected with MRSA can safely be cared for in residential and nursing homes, as well as in their own homes[56], and seminars have been held for managers of residential and nursing homes, their insurers and staff responsible for their statutory registration.

Reliable data on the epidemiology of infections are essential to inform the targeting of resources to control them. New guidance on hospital infection control, issued in March 1995, includes a chapter on improving the surveillance of hospital-acquired infections, with specific advice on antibiotic-resistant organisms[57]. In October 1995, DH funded the Public Health Laboratory Service to develop a national nosocomial infection surveillance scheme.

But MRSA are by no means the only bacteria in which the emergence of antibiotic resistance is a cause for concern. Aminoglycoside- and cephalosporin-resistant *Klebsiellae* and vancomycin-resistant *Enterococci* are being identified with increasing frequency, and have caused outbreaks in hospitals. These organisms mainly affect patients in intensive care and other specialised units, particularly patients who are immunocompromised. Penicillin-resistant *Pneumococci* are now being isolated from cases of community-acquired pneumonia, and resistant strains of *Salmonellae* are also increasingly seen. A Working Group of the ACMSF has been established to review the role of food in the acquisition of infection with antibiotic-resistant micro-organisms and the need for action to protect public health. Multidrug-resistant strains of *Mycobacterium tuberculosis* are still uncommon in the UK, but have caused outbreaks recently in two London hospitals[58,59]; guidance on the prevention and control of infection due to such strains, and of HIV-related tuberculosis, is expected to be published in 1996.

Information technology

Information technology (IT) and the use of computers has revolutionised the way in which patient care is delivered and health improved. Rapid developments indicate that, over the next few years, the pace of change will become even faster, providing greater potential benefits to patients and the public, with likely improvements in public health, health care, education, research and management effectiveness. However, there are also potential disadvantages in the process and, in particular, a need to maintain the confidentiality of individual patient information.

Public health can be improved by the introduction of information technology. Intelligence systems can be refined and provide rapid warning of changes in patterns of health, with increased computational power allowing new and more effective epidemiological investigations to improve the quality of data and its predictive value. The ability to generate large databases on health issues allows patterns of illness and disease to be more clearly delineated, and causes identified; coupled with the use of geographical information systems, the ability to map disease is thereby enhanced. For environmental health and communicable diseases, such facilities are invaluable and can lead both to better control of a problem, and to a better understanding of its pathogenesis.

Patient care is already enhanced by the use of computers. In this country, there are already high levels of computer use in hospitals and general practices. The further development of the electronic patient record and integrated clinical workstations will improve this even further. The technology available at the bedside, in the laboratory, and through satellite links with the advent of telemedicine shows how the care of individual patients can be improved. The use of IT for clinical audit and assessment of effectiveness of care and in evidence-based care programmes allows the best care to be delivered to individual patients. Multi-media and telemedicine developments enable a wide range of clinical information to be exchanged. For example, information from diagnostic systems, radiological procedures, laboratory tests, and cardiological and videotape evidence can all be transmitted to almost anywhere in the world for expert advice; ambulance systems using computers and geographical information systems can track vehicles and direct them most effectively to where they are needed most; and drug interactions and treatment protocols can readily be made available.

From an educational point of view, patients and professionals alike can benefit. Patients can more readily gain access to information via the Internet or by specially designed facilities in hospital or primary care. They can be helped to ask questions and participate more fully in their own care, and it becomes easier to discuss the range of treatment options available and the results of therapy and possible adverse reactions. The development of 'smart cards' may allow better integration and sharing of care. From the professional perspective, computer-assisted learning can allow greater degrees of personally directed learning packages; access to databases and evidence for effectiveness enable clinicians to update information and to improve communication with patients; technical advances in the use of IT can improve patient care and allow exploration of new methods of treatment; and research methodologies can be greatly expanded.

The use of IT also allows for improvement in the management of the health service, making it easier to provide and analyse services, and to plan them more effectively, taking account of local needs, patients' perspectives and clinical outcomes, and allowing the delivery of health care to be more effectively integrated.

There is excitement in IT's possibilities of allowing improved care to patients, and the potential is enormous. However, there are disadvantages, including the need for patients, professionals and managers to understand the implications and to ensure that they are adequately trained; a culture change is required. However, the main concern, for all interest groups, is the issue of patient confidentiality. Trust between patient and doctor has been at the heart of medical practice for centuries. Codes of ethics and guidance from regulatory bodies such as the General Medical Council (GMC) have set out the principles involved. DH has also published guidance on this subject[60]. The principles have not altered; what has changed is the potential ability to gain access to large amounts of personal information by use of computers rather then in a paper-based form. This is an issue which must be treated with all seriousness. It requires full public debate and effective dialogue between those parties most concerned. The consultation between a patient and a doctor is integral to delivery of health care; the processes in place now, and in the future, must not jeopardise this relationship.

HIV infection and AIDS

The cause of AIDS, first clinically recognised in the early 1980s, was initially unknown but was attributed to a deficiency of the immune system. The voluntary surveillance system in England (co-ordinated by the Communicable Disease Surveillance Centre of the Public Health Laboratory Service) started in 1982 and three AIDS cases were reported, increasing to 24 in 1983, 73 in 1984 and 151 in 1985. HIV was isolated and characterised in 1983, and the subsequent development of serological tests allowed the detection of infection before symptoms appeared and enabled testing of blood and tissue donations to protect the public health. The rapid spread of AIDS among homosexual men in the United States of America, with an increase in reported cases here, raised serious concerns about how the epidemic might develop and what action should be taken. The Department had very limited data initially but prompt establishment of information campaigns warned the public about the epidemic and ensured that the UK remained a country with a relatively low prevalence of infection. The identification of this novel communicable disease, the aetiology and natural history of which were at first unknown, has provided valuable lessons for the role of epidemiology and preventive medicine in the protection of the general population, and particular groups at increased risk, until research studies can establish the true nature of a novel disease.

Since the 1980s, detailed information on sexual behaviour from the National Survey of Sexual Attitudes and Lifestyles and information from the unlinked anonymous surveys on trends in prevalence have become available (see page 156). Together with the reports of AIDS cases and HIV infections, these data have provided a more detailed picture of HIV infection in the UK. It has now been estimated that, in 1993, 22,900 adults were infected with HIV in England and Wales. Improved surveillance has also helped to provide more accurate projections of the epidemic. Latest data indicate that nearly 7,000 people were living with AIDS or other forms of severe HIV disease, and this figure is projected to increase to over 8,000 by the end of the decade. The epidemic is still largely confined to particular groups, with homosexual and bisexual men being the largest component; however, incidence among heterosexuals is projected to increase. Since HIV was first isolated and identified, research has provided much information about transmission and pathogenesis of HIV - but there is still much more to learn. Results from carefully controlled clinical trials have provided information on various treatment regimens, but a cure or a vaccine are still not available. Surveillance systems to monitor the epidemic continue to be developed to underpin health education campaigns; control of HIV/AIDS still depends on effective health promotion messages to the general population and to those most vulnerable to infection.

EXECUTIVE SUMMARY

VITAL STATISTICS

Population size

The estimated resident population of England at 30 June 1995 was 48.9 million, a 0.4% increase compared with 1994.

Age and sex structure of the resident population

The number of children below school age remains fairly stable. The population of school-age children continues to increase slowly. The younger working population aged 16-29 years is falling, whereas the older working population (aged 30-59 years for women and 30-64 years for men) is increasing. The most elderly group of pensioners (aged 85 years and over) continues to increase and represents a growing proportion of all pensioners.

Fertility statistics - aspects of relevance for health care

In 1993, 776,800 conceptions occurred to women resident in England, a 1% fall from the figure in 1992, with an overall provisional conception rate of 76.3 per 1,000 women aged 15-44 years. In 1995, there were 613,257 live births in England - 2.5% fewer than in 1994, and the fifth successive year to show a fall. In 1994, 149,764 abortions were performed on women resident in England, a fall of 0.8% compared with 1993.

Mortality

Deaths registered in England increased from 517,614 in 1994 to 529,038 in 1995, a rise of 2.2%, but fewer than the 541,121 deaths registered in 1993. For most age-groups, mortality rates fell during the 1980s in males and females, but a 7.5% increase was seen for men aged 15-44 years between 1985 and 1990; the mortality rate among men in this age-group fell between 1990 and 1993, but was 5% higher in 1995 than in 1985.

Prevalence of disease in the community

Figures from the General Practice Research Database in 1994 show that 6.4% of the population were prescribed asthma drugs and had a diagnosis of asthma; 9.8% of women and 4.1% of men aged 16 years and over had a diagnosis of depression and had been prescribed antidepressants; and 11.7% of men and 9.2% of women aged 35 years and over had a diagnosis of hypertension and had been treated with antihypertensive drugs.

In 1994, 32% of respondents to the General Household Survey (GHS)[61] reported a long-standing illness, 19% a limiting long-standing illness, and 14% restricted activity during the two weeks before interview. The proportion of the population with a limiting long-term illness may vary between different ethnic groups and geographical area, according to data from the 1991 Census.

Infant and perinatal mortality

Provisional statistics for 1995 in England indicate that 3,721 babies died before the age of one year, compared with 3,861 in 1994. The infant mortality rate remained at 6.1 per 1,000 live-births, the lowest ever recorded. There were 3,406 stillbirths in 1995 compared with 3,584 in 1994; the stillbirth rate fell to 5.5 per 1,000 total births.

Trends in cancer incidence and mortality

Data from the 1988[62] and 1989[63] GHSs show that 1% of adults reported cancer as a cause for long-standing illness, and a similar figure is indicated by the Office of Population Censuses and Surveys (OPCS)/Office for National Statistics (ONS) Longitudinal Study. There was an increase in incidence for all malignant neoplasms combined (excluding non-melanoma skin cancer) between 1979 and 1991. Registrations of malignant melanoma of the skin rose considerably for men and women over this period. When adjusted for age, lung cancer registration rates fell for males but increased for females between 1979 and 1991.

Trends in reporting congenital anomalies

According to provisional data for 1995, the rate for malformed live births fell to 80.7 per 10,000 live births, 1% lower than in 1994 and 28% lower than in 1990.

THE NATION'S HEALTH

Recent health trends in England

Substantial reductions in mortality rates have occurred over the last 25 years: adjusted for age differences, mortality rates have fallen by about 30% since 1970. Nevertheless, mortality rates for coronary heart disease (CHD) and cancers remain relatively high compared with other European Union (EU) countries. The Health Survey for England[64,65] is a major part of a wider Department of Health (DH) survey programme to monitor the health of the population.

Inter-Departmental Group on Public Health

The Inter-Departmental Group on Public Health, chaired by the Chief Medical Officer, facilitates discussion and exchange of information on health issues across a wide range of Government Departments.

Variations in health

The Chief Medical Officer set up a Working Group to look at what DH and the National Health Service (NHS) could do to tackle social class, gender, geographical and ethnic variations in health in the Health of the Nation key areas[1]. The Group reported in October[33].

Housing and health

Housing conditions can contribute to ill-health, but complex interactions with a number of other factors mean that it is often difficult to assess the individual effect of any one possible cause.

Substance misuse

Sensible drinking[66], a review of the health effects of drinking alcohol, was published in December. Work continues nationally and locally to pursue the Government's anti-drugs strategy as set out in *Tackling drugs together*[38]. The Department launched the National Drugs Helpline and provided £1 million to develop drugs services for young people.

Nutrition

The Nutrition Task Force published nutritional guidelines for hospital catering[67] and, with the Physical Activity Task Force, a report on obesity[68]. The Committee on Medical Aspects of Food and Nutrition Policy (COMA) set up two working groups on nutritional assessment of modifications to infant formulas and on dietary intakes and nutritional status with regard to folic acid and to nutrients currently added to flour and yellow fats. The report of a nutrition survey of children aged $1^1/_2$ to $4^1/_2$ years was published[69].

Health of children

During 1995, the distinct health needs of children were further recognised, particularly in the Health of the Young Nation initiative. The Health Select Committee announced an inquiry into children's health[70].

Health of adolescents

In July, Ministers launched the Health of the Young Nation initiative, which focuses the Government's strategy for health[1] on young people. Health-related behaviours and effective health promotion for young people have been identified as priority areas for research, which will be assisted by the projected multidisciplinary National Adolescent Health Network.

Health of women

Women's health was highlighted in September at the Fourth United Nations (UN) World Conference on Women, and a UK implementation plan was announced for the global platform for action.

Health of men

Men's health issues are increasingly emphasised, with a wide range of projects and events to improve the impact of health promotion messages for men.

Health of black and ethnic minorities

Work to improve the health of black and ethnic minorities continues to be developed within DH and the NHS. The analysis of the ethnicity question in the 1991 Census data will provide better information to understand the needs of ethnic minority populations.

Health in the workplace

The new Reporting of Injuries, Diseases and Dangerous Occurrences Regulations (RIDDOR) 1995[71] will come into force on 1 April 1996. The Health and Safety Executive (HSE) and OPCS, in collaboration with independent experts, published the *Occupational Health Decennial Supplement*[72], and in May the HSE launched its occupational health campaign 'Good health is good business'.

Health of people in later life

DH continued to promote work on sickness and disability prevention for older people, and to promote services to facilitate independent life in the community. Guidance was issued on NHS responsibilities for meeting continuing health care needs[73], and local policies and criteria will come into operation in 1996.

THE STRATEGY FOR HEALTH

Introduction

The Health of the Nation strategy[1] continues to influence the development of health services and initiatives to improve health, whether generated by DH, the NHS or other Government Departments and non-Governmental organisations. In July, DH published *Fit for the future*[74], the second progress report on the strategy. The conference to mark the third anniversary of the strategy for health also launched the Health of the Young Nation initiative.

Key areas and targets

Coronary heart disease and stroke: Action to achieve targets focused on physical activity, obesity and serum cholesterol concentrations. The Health Survey for England for 1993[65], published in 1995, focused on CHD and associated risk-factors. The Stroke Health Outcomes Group met for the first time in December; its remit is to develop indicators which will contribute to policy on health interventions and the planning of services.

Cancers: Early detection through screening continues to be the key intervention for breast and cervical cancers. Work to reduce skin cancer incidence has concentrated on increasing public awareness of the dangers of over-exposing the skin to ultraviolet radiation and encouraging everyone to take sensible precautions in the sun. Adult cigarette smoking rates continued to fall, but rates among schoolchildren rose. A television campaign was launched as part of the Government's three-year anti-smoking campaign.

Mental illness: Work has focused on development and use of measures of health strategy targets and related issues. The OPCS was commissioned to carry out the first national survey of psychiatric morbidity. Mental health became one of the six priorities in the *Priorities and planning guidance* for the NHS[34].

HIV/AIDS and sexual health: DH allocated £244.7 million in 1995/96 to health authorities towards HIV treatment costs, including £49 million to help to prevent the spread of HIV infection. Conceptions among girls aged under 16 years are now falling.

Accidents: There continues to be good progress towards the accident targets[1]. The Accident Prevention Task Force has commissioned and distributed a number of reports, and inter-Departmental working has contributed to the success of various safety initiatives, including Child Safety Week.

Variations in health

The Chief Medical Officer set up a Working Group to look at what DH and the NHS could do to tackle social class, gender, geographical and ethnic variations in health in the Health of the Nation key areas[1,33].

Implementation

Priorities for the NHS: The strategy for health continues to provide the main context for NHS planning. The NHS Executive is developing a performance management framework with Regional Offices and health authorities. The Executive has a project team to provide practical help and support to the NHS in implementing the strategy.

Local health alliances: In its first year, the Health Alliance Awards Scheme attracted over 300 entries, most of a high standard. The Scheme includes a special category for projects relevant to the Health of the Young Nation for 1995/96, its second year.

Healthy settings: Work on healthy settings involves many other Government Departments. DH is developing closer links with the UK Health For All Network.

Inter-Departmental co-operation: Led by a Cabinet sub-Committee, Government Departments are pursuing various initiatives which contribute to the Health of the Nation initiative.

The way ahead

As a long-term strategy, the Health of the Nation initiative needs to be underpinned by robust data. During 1996, DH will publish an overview of behavioural epidemiology to contribute to the understanding of health-related behaviours.

MENTAL HEALTH

Introduction

DH has set an evidence-based mental health strategy which encompasses where and how people with mental illness are cared for, and why. The Health of the Nation strategy[1] sets targets for mental illness; the framework to improve health and social outcomes and reduce mortality involves the improvement of information and understanding, the development of comprehensive local services, and the general encouragement of good practice.

Information about mental illness

Monitoring the state of public mental health, planning the nature and volumes of services likely to be required and evaluating the effectiveness of services provided all depend on reliable information. In the light of the Health of the Nation targets[1], and the broader aims they reflect, the scope and nature of information collection about disorders in the general population, in primary care and in secondary care is being comprehensively reviewed and upgraded.

Epidemiology of mental disorders: An extensive two-phase epidemiological survey of psychiatric morbidity throughout Great Britain has been carried out by the OPCS and an advisory group of psychiatric epidemiologists in samples from households, institutions and among homeless people[75,76,77,78,79,80,81,82]. This is the first national survey in any country to collect data on prevalence, risk-factors, and associated disability simultaneously in household, institutional and homeless samples by use of standardised assessment techniques. One in seven adults aged 16 to 64 years who are living in private households had suffered from some type of neurotic disorder in the week before the survey interview, half of which was mixed anxiety-depressive disorder. All types of neurotic disorders were more common among women than men. Subjects with significant depressive symptoms were asked about suicidal ideas. Just under 1% of the total sample in the OPCS survey reported suicidal thoughts in the preceding week, two-thirds of them women. One-fifth of those reporting suicidal ideas were receiving antidepressant medication and one-sixth were receiving counselling or psychotherapy. One adult in 20 had experienced symptoms of alcohol dependence in the preceding year and one in 40 dependence on drugs. Functional psychoses carry an even higher likelihood than neuroses of a chronic disabling course, and thus incidence and prevalence differ considerably. The OPCS national survey indicated that the overall prevalence of psychosis (mainly schizophrenia and affective disorders) was four per 1,000, with that for urban dwellers being twice that for those living in the country. Of people with psychosis, two-thirds had been in touch with specialist services, whilst 18% had seen only their GP in the year before interview and a further 18% claimed never to have sought professional help.

Mental disorders in primary care: A recent World Health Organization (WHO) international collaborative study of mental health in primary care showed that well-defined psychological problems are common in all primary care settings (about 24% of all consultations)[83]. This finding is borne out by local studies[84].

Information about specialist mental health services: Statistics about the activity of specialist mental health services in the NHS have been collected by DH for many years[85] to support policy development, strategic planning, the security and allocation of resources, and performance management. In view of developments in the approach to the management of people with chronic and severe mental disorders living in the community, and the need to collect information to monitor Health of the Nation targets[1], the Department is considering a revision of the framework for national mental health statistics to produce a system which reflects the complex multidisciplinary care arranged for such patients, including that provided outwith the NHS, and which is useful to clinical staff for clinical purposes. Issues of confidentiality and data security will be critical.

Measuring mental health outcomes: A key feature of the new mental health Data Set will be the Health of the Nation Outcome Scale (HoNOS)[47,48].

Confidential Inquiry into Homicides and Suicides by Mentally Ill People: Two Health of the Nation targets[1] relate to suicides. A Confidential Inquiry into Homicides and Suicides by Mentally Ill People was established in 1992 and the first of two reports appeared this year[86,87].

Research and development in mental health: The Department's Research and Development (R&D) Directorate oversees two complementary research programmes which include mental health initiatives.

Public information strategy: The Government has set up a three-year public information strategy to influence public attitudes to mental health services, which aims to increase understanding, reduce stigma and help users to understand both their rights and responsibilities.

Development of services for mental health care

A local comprehensive mental health and learning disability service strategy needs to address the needs of children, adults and older people in the general population in primary care, in secondary care, in specialist tertiary care, in prisons and among other groups such as the homeless.

Children and adolescents: DH has commissioned several research projects into child and adolescent mental health services (CAMHS). The *Handbook on child and adolescent mental health*[88] was followed by the Health Advisory Service's review *Together we stand*[89].

Adults with mental health problems: A wide range of mental disorders is seen in primary care settings. A recent survey[83] indicated that one-quarter of consecutive attenders at GP surgeries had at least one, and 14% had at least two, mental ill-health diagnoses. The commonest was depression (17%), followed by anxiety states and panic disorder (11% each), chronic fatigue (10%) and alcohol-related problems (4%).

Adults with severe mental illness: In August, the Minister for Health asked NHS regional directors to review the progress made in their regions towards the delivery of modern and effective mental health services. Although the results of that review, to be published in February 1996, showed that every health authority now has a strategic plan for fully comprehensive local services, many still had progress to make towards achieving them. These will continue to be monitored until fully implemented. The care programme approach (CPA)[90] was introduced in 1991 to ensure: services assess needs for health and social care; a package of care is assembled to meet those needs, drawn up in agreement with the multidisciplinary health team, social services, GPs, user and carers; a key worker is appointed to keep close contact with the patient; and that regular review and monitoring of the patient's needs and progress, and of the delivery of care, takes place. The CPA is tiered, so that patients with the greatest needs receive the most comprehensive package of care. Supervision registers[91] were introduced to identify patients who are at significant risk of suicide, serious harm to others or serious self-neglect. They are a flexible and temporary priority listing of those on the CPA who are considered most at risk.

People with learning disabilities: In the period since the White Paper *Better services for the mentally handicapped*[92], care and support for people with learning disabilities has shifted towards an approach based on individual needs. In common with the rest of the population, people with learning disabilities have physical and emotional needs that will be provided by a normal and healthy lifestyle. During 1994-95, the Social Services Inspectorate (SSI) mounted an inspection of leisure and recreation facilities in day-care services[93]; a national development team has been commissioned to produce a handbook based on the experiences of hospital closure; and research was commissioned to evaluate various types of non-hospital accommodation and support.

Older people with mental health problems: GPs retain their roles as gatekeepers to specialist multidisciplinary old age psychiatry services, but with the implementation of the NHS and Community Care Act 1990[94] social services now purchase most continuing support for older people with mental health problems. The major mental health problems for older people are dementias and affective disorders; the diagnosis of both can be difficult in old age.

The way ahead

Besides ensuring that the core elements of a local comprehensive service are in place in every health authority, with particular attention to mental health needs in areas of high deprivation in inner cities, it is important to pay attention to mental health promotion, the development and introduction of clinical practice guidelines, an improved interface between primary and secondary care, suicide prevention, collaboration with industry to ensure a healthy working population, and international co-operation in research and service development.

Mental health promotion: Primary prevention is intended to prevent the onset of mental disorder; secondary prevention to detect and treat mental disorder early; and tertiary prevention to maintain the health and social functioning of people with a diagnosed mental disorder[95].

Clinical practice guidelines: The Royal College of Psychiatrists and the Department are working together to explore ways to implement clinical practice guidelines through continuing medical education and through performance management of purchasing by local health authorities.

Suicide prevention: Suicide prevention needs to: reduce access to means; increase public awareness; target high-risk groups; and develop primary and secondary care[96,97].

Ensuring a healthy workforce: Studies of minor psychiatric morbidity in working populations indicate a high prevalence of between 27-37%[98]. Minor psychiatric disorder is a major determinant of sickness absence, and is the second most common cause of prolonged absence. Within the workplace, people suffering from mental health problems may work less effectively and their relationships with colleagues and customers may be impaired.

International links: DH's mental health division maintains close collaboration with the WHO and with mental health policy-makers around the world.

Mental health into the 21st Century: Mental health has long been regarded as a mysterious, enigmatic, difficult and even frightening topic. Mental health should be valued as much as physical health, and health policies and initiatives in the workplace and schools, as well as in the NHS, ought to include a proper focus on mental health.

HEALTH CARE

Role and function of the National Health Service in England

Strategic purpose: The purpose of the National Health Service (NHS) is to secure through the resources available the greatest possible improvement to the physical and mental health of the people of England by: promoting health, preventing ill-health, diagnosing and treating disease and injury, and caring for those with long-term illness and disability who require the services of the NHS - a service available to all on the basis of clinical need, regardless of the ability to pay. In seeking to achieve this purpose as a public service, the NHS aims to judge its results under three headings - equity, efficiency and responsiveness.

Policies: The main Government policies for meeting the purpose of the NHS and for delivering these results are set out in the Health of the Nation White Paper[1], *Caring for people*[99] and *The patient's charter*[100], and in moves towards a primary care-led NHS.

27

Priority setting: The overall context for the planning and delivery of NHS services is set out in the annual *Priorities and planning guidance*[34]. Health authorities and GP fundholders assess the needs of the people they serve and decide which treatments and services are required to meet those needs, and individual clinicians decide on the most clinically appropriate treatment for their patients.

Research and development: The research and development (R&D) strategy has two complementary programmes: the policy research programme, which provides a knowledge base for strategic matters across the Department and provides evidence-based findings which advance Health of the Nation objectives[1]; and the NHS R&D strategy, which is priority led with a key role in evidence-based health care. An information systems strategy advances the dissemination of research findings. Work continues to take forward implementation of the Culyer Task Force recommendations[101]. The House of Lords report on medical research[102,103] warmly welcomed the R&D achievements of the Department.

Role of the NHS in maintaining public health

Public health and the NHS: *Public health in England*[104], published in July 1994, outlined the public health functions of health authorities. All health authorities are required to make arrangements to involve professionals in the full range of their work.

'Making it happen': Publication of the report *Making it happen*[105] sets out recommendations about the crucial role that nursing professionals can play in promoting public health.

Health needs assessment: The assessment of health needs continued to develop as a core activity of District Health Authorities (DHAs).

National confidential enquiries: Reports were published by the National Confidential Enquiry into Peri-operative Deaths (NCEPOD)[106] and the Confidential Enquiry into Stillbirths and Deaths in Infancy (CESDI)[107].

National Casemix Office and NHS Centre for Coding and Classification: Work progressed to develop health care terms (from Read Codes), classifications and groupings of patient level data to support resource management and needs assessment.

Quality of service and effectiveness of care: The delivery of effective health care services must reflect an up-to-date knowledge and understanding of current research.

Clinical and health outcomes: The Central Health Outcomes Unit (CHOU) has an extensive programme to develop outcome indicators, and supports various projects which aim to develop the methods and information options necessary to create new indicators.

Regional epidemiological services for communicable disease: Surveillance, prevention and control of communicable disease remains a fundamental public health task. A national Service Level Agreement with the Public Health Laboratory Service (PHLS) was signed in November and will come into effect on 1 April 1996.

Primary health care

Organisation of primary care: Changes in the organisation of primary care have enabled improvements in inter-professional care, more effective working practices for GPs and more efficient, and often more local, provision of services to patients.

Prescribing: Costs of GP prescribing continue to rise faster than other NHS spending. However, further progress in quality and cost-effectiveness was also seen, and developments in information technology and involvement of other health care professionals should help to maintain this progress.

Professional development and clinical audit: Clinical audit and continuing professional development now include evidence-based audit protocols and training for personal and practice development planning and review.

Specialised clinical services

Specialised services: Developments in specialised clinical services should lead to improved services to patients.

Cancer: In April, after wide consultation, a strategic framework for the future development of cancer services was unveiled, based on the report of an Expert Advisory Group on cancer[108].

Minimal access therapy: Training facilities opened at the Royal College of Surgeons of England and Leeds already have well established courses.

Osteoporosis: Ministers endorsed the report of the Advisory Group on Osteoporosis[109].

Transplantation: The Advisory Group on the Ethics of Xenotransplantation started work in December and will report to the Secretary of State for Health during Summer, 1996.

Strategic Review of Pathology Services: The report of the Strategic Review of Pathology Services was published in September[110].

Intensive care: Guidelines were prepared on admissions to and discharges from intensive-care and high-dependency units, and will be issued in Spring, 1996.

Emergency admissions: The increase in emergency admissions, with considerable local variations, posed challenges for the management of hospital workloads.

Maternity and child health services

Implementation of 'Changing Childbirth': The second year of the five-year implementation schedule was completed, with good progress being made. The Implementation Team established itself as a source of advice and support, and work on monitoring progress began.

Folic acid and prevention of neural tube defects: In June, DH awarded a contract to the HEA to run a folic acid awareness campaign over the next 2^1/$_2$ years. An Expert Group will be set up by the COMA to assess and report on the health aspects of increasing folate/folic acid intakes.

Sudden infant death syndrome: Mortality from sudden infant death syndrome (SIDS) remained at the rate of 0.6 per 1,000 live births in 1994, a fall of more than 70% compared with 1988 figures.

Prophylaxis of vitamin K deficiency bleeding in infants: This subject was kept under review and research findings are expected to be published during 1996.

Retinopathy of prematurity: A report of progress on a nationwide research, training and audit programme began.

Paediatric intensive care: Research on issues related to paediatric intensive care is being incorporated in the NHS R&D programme to provide more data about factors which influence the survival of critically ill children.

Congenital anomalies: A report was published by the working group set up by the Medical Advisory Committee of the Registrar General of the OPCS[111].

Asthma

DH and others organised a conference in November on the possible causes and successful management of asthma. A new NHS research and development strategy was launched on asthma management.

Diabetes mellitus

The final report of the joint DH/British Diabetic Association St Vincent Task Force for Diabetes was published[112].

Complementary medicine

Progress continued towards implementation of the statutory regulation of osteopaths and chiropractors. Research indicates that 40% of GP practices provide access to some form of complementary therapy for NHS patients[113].

Disability and rehabilitation

Further developments included a series of co-ordinated initiatives on epilepsy, incontinence, pressure sore prevention, brain rehabilitation projects and refinement of target setting.

Prison health care

A national drugs strategy was launched to reduce supply of and demand for substances liable to misuse and to improve rehabilitation[114].

COMMUNICABLE DISEASES

HIV infection and AIDS

HIV infection and AIDS data showed a similar pattern to previous years. A summary of AIDS projections for England and Wales until 1999[115] forecast that the overall incidence of AIDS cases was expected to level off in 1996 and 1997, but that there would be underlying differences in trends between exposure categories. AIDS incidence among homosexual males, the numerically largest group, may fall. The incidence among those exposed heterosexually or by intravenous drug misuse was expected to increase gradually.

Other sexually transmitted diseases

The total number of new cases seen at genito-urinary medicine clinics continues to rise. New gonorrhoea cases fell by 2% in 1994 and the rate of 37 per 100,000 is below the Health of the Nation target of 49 per 100,000 population by the year 1995[1]. Reports of new cases of *Chlamydia trachomatis* and first attacks of herpes simplex virus rose.

Immunisation

Immunisation coverage, apart from measles, mumps, rubella (MMR) vaccine, continues to rise; 95% coverage targets have been met by the child's second birthday for the other childhood vaccines. The impact of the 1994 measles, rubella immunisation campaign is now apparent. Measles cases are at exceptionally low levels, and a number of the confirmed cases have been shown to be imported. A routine second dose of MMR vaccine has been recommended for all eligible children at the time of the pre-school boosters of diphtheria, tetanus and polio vaccines.

Viral hepatitis

Viral hepatitis is a notifiable disease. In 1995, a provisional total of 3,156 cases were notified to the OPCS from England; of these, 2,043 were due to hepatitis A and 599 due to hepatitis B.

Influenza

Two peaks of influenza activity occurred during 1995, in February and December.

Meningitis

There was a considerable increase in meningococcal infection in 1995 with a shift towards more Group C disease, more septicaemic features at presentation, and with more older children affected. Nevertheless, case-fatality rates appear to have fallen.

Tuberculosis

Notifications of tuberculosis showed signs of levelling out again in 1995 following the small year-on-year increases at the beginning of the decade. New guidance on tuberculosis control was completed, for publication in 1996.

Hospital-acquired infection

New guidance on hospital infection control was issued in March[116]. Methicillin-resistant *Staphylococcus aureus* continued to cause outbreaks of infection in hospitals.

Foodborne and waterborne diseases

Notifications of food poisoning to the OPCS in 1995 were little different from those for 1994. Similarly, the number of laboratory isolations of *Campylobacter* and *Salmonella* remained virtually unchanged from last year, although isolations of *Salmonella typhimurium* definitive type (DT) 104 continue to increase and are being investigated. Reports of human listeriosis showed a fall of 19%. Verocytotoxin-producing *Escherichia coli* (VTEC) O157 showed a 93% increase over the previous year, although this increase may be related partly to improved ascertainment following publication during the year of the Advisory Committee on the Microbiological Safety of Food's report on VTEC[29]. A large outbreak of cryptosporidiosis thought likely to be associated with water occurred in Devon.

Emerging infectious diseases

In response to international concern about the threat from new and re-emerging infectious diseases, the WHO established a new Division of Emerging and other Communicable Diseases Surveillance and Control.

Travel-related disease

The new book *Health information for overseas travel*, which draws together health information for doctors and other health professionals who advise travellers, was published[117]. An outbreak of Legionnaires' disease associated with a Turkish hotel highlighted the need for greater awareness of this disease among operators in the travel industry.

ENVIRONMENTAL HEALTH AND TOXICOLOGY

Chemical and physical agents in the environment

Small Area Health Statistics Unit: The Small Area Health Statistics Unit investigates claims of unusual clusters of disease or ill-health in the vicinity of point sources of pollution from chemicals and/or radiation.

Air pollution: Reports on the effects on health of airborne particles[118] and on the relation between asthma and air pollution[119] were published during the year, as well as a report on the effects on health of exposures to mixtures of pollutants[120]. Two further recommendations for air quality standards, for particles and sulphur dioxide, were made.

Committee on Medical Aspects of Radiation in the Environment: The Committee published a joint report with the Radioactive Waste Management Advisory Committee on potential health effects and possible sources of radioactive particles found in the vicinity of the Dounreay nuclear establishment[121].

Environment and health: DH continued to participate nationally and internationally in activities to identify, and protect against, risks to public health from environmental factors.

Surveillance of diseases possibly due to non-infectious environmental hazards: Work is in progress to improve the ability to respond to possible health effects of non-infectious hazards in the environment.

Toxicological safety

Food chemical hazards: The Committee on Toxicity of Chemicals in Food, Consumer Products and the Environment continued to provide independent expert advice, including confirmation of its earlier assessment on dioxins[122,123], which occur as contaminants in food, and on the acceptability of the sweetener, cyclamate.

Potential chemical carcinogens: The Committee on Carcinogenicity of Chemicals in Food, Consumer Products and the Environment reviewed animal studies on the effects of the insecticide carbaryl, and its advice led to restrictions being placed on the use of carbaryl in pesticidal products and in human medicines to control head lice[124].

Traditional and herbal remedies: New legislation maintained previous controls on herbal remedies. The cause of the few possible cases where adverse reactions may have occurred was often uncertain.

33

Novel foods: The Advisory Committee on Novel Foods and Processes evaluated a wide range of novel foods, including a starter culture used to produce cultured milk products, several genetically modified crop plants used to produce processed food ingredients (oilseed rape and maize) and a genetically modified tomato to be eaten fresh.

Pesticides: DH continued to advise on pesticide safety and was involved in revision of UK pesticide approvals to meet the demands of the new European Union (EU) system for authorisation of plant protection products.

Veterinary products: DH continued to provide advice to the Ministry of Agriculture, Fisheries and Food on the human safety aspects of veterinary products and animal feeds. The Department is jointly funding an epidemiological study into the health of sheep dippers and has drawn doctors' attention to this topic[125].

MEDICAL EDUCATION, TRAINING AND STAFFING

Junior doctors' hours

'New Deal' monitoring arrangements were strengthened during the year. The September reporting round showed 93% compliance with the 1996 targets for contracted hours. Action to reduce actual hours of work and work intensity remains a priority.

Advisory Group on Medical and Dental Education, Training and Staffing and the Specialist Workforce Advisory Group

The Advisory Group on Medical and Dental Education, Training and Staffing (AGMETS), which advises Ministers on medical and dental education, training and staffing matters, met four times during 1995. The Specialist Workforce Advisory Group (SWAG) was set up in the early part of the year, and met representatives of all medical specialties as part of the process of advising on the required numbers of doctors in higher specialist training.

Medical Workforce Standing Advisory Committee

The Government has accepted the Medical Workforce Standing Advisory Committee's recommendation[126] to increase medical school intake by 500 to 4,970 by the year 2000.

Postgraduate and specialist medical education

Implementation of *Hospital doctors: training for the future*[127] (the Calman Report) started during 1995. The necessary legislation for these specialist medical training reforms, the European Specialist Medical Qualifications Order 1995[128], will come into force on 12 January 1996. A major strand of these reforms is the introduction of a unified higher specialist training grade. The new specialist registrar grade was launched in December in two specialties, general surgery and diagnostic radiology, and all other specialties will follow in a year-long rolling programme starting on 1 April 1996. The training reforms are on course for full implementation by the year 2000. Important changes for the management of postgraduate medical and dental education were also set in place.

Equal opportunities for doctors and the part-time consultants scheme

Continued progress was made during the year to encourage equal opportunities for doctors. In particular, steps were taken to ensure reasonable opportunities for flexible training as part of the preparations for the launch of the new specialist registrar grade.

Undergraduate medical and dental education

The Steering Group on Undergraduate Medical and Dental Education and Research has reviewed arrangements for liaison between the NHS and universities following the Health Authorities Act 1995[129], and its recommendations will be published in early 1996. New arrangements for the Service Increment for Teaching (SIFT) were agreed during 1995, and will take effect from 1 April 1996.

Medical (Professional Performance) Act

The Medical (Professional Performance) Act 1995[130] was enacted in November. The General Medical Council (GMC) is now developing detailed procedures with a view to the Act coming into force in 1997.

Maintaining medical excellence

The report *Maintaining medical excellence*[131] was published in August. It emphasises the need to ensure and improve the quality and delivery of health care by supporting doctors to maintain high standards. A key recommendation is for the introduction of mentoring systems for all hospital medical staff. Much of this work will require the close collaboration and support of NHS managers, practising doctors, professional organisations and all those involved in medical education.

Locum doctors

The Working Group on Hospital Locum Doctors published a report for consultation in January[132].

OTHER TOPICS OF INTEREST IN 1995

Medicines Control Agency

Role and performance: The role of the Medicines Control Agency (MCA) is to protect public health by ensuring that all medicines for human use meet stringent criteria of safety, quality and efficacy. The MCA met almost all of its key targets during the year.

Legal reclassification of medicinal products: During 1995, two substances were reclassified as prescription medicines, five were reclassified to allow sale from pharmacies, and two were reclassified for general sale.

Oral contraceptives: In October, following a special meeting convened to consider findings of three studies, the Committee on Safety of Medicines recommended that oral contraceptives (OCs) containing desogestrel or gestodene should only be used by women who are intolerant of other combined OCs and prepared to accept an increased risk of thromboembolism[42].

Pharmaceutical developments in the European Union: The MCA played a leading role in the operation of the new EU marketing authorisation system.

European Medicines Evaluation Agency

The European Medicines Evaluation Agency has been established in London's Docklands to support the new EU marketing authorisation procedures which came into force on 1 January.

Medical Devices Agency

The Medical Devices Agency is an Executive Agency of DH. Its role is to ensure that all medical devices and equipment used in the UK meet appropriate standards of safety, quality and performance. The Agency achieves this role through implementation of the EU Medical Devices Directives, a reporting system for device-related adverse incidents, an evaluation programme of a wide range of medical devices and the publication of safety and advice information.

National Blood Authority

In November, Ministers accepted the National Blood Authority's proposals for the future organisation of the national blood service. An independent national user group will monitor delivery of service to hospitals. An interim Blood Donor's Charter has been introduced[133].

National Biological Standards Board

The National Biological Standards Board has a statutory duty to assure the quality of biological substances used in medicine.

National Radiological Protection Board

The National Radiological Protection Board was set up to acquire and advance knowledge about the protection of mankind from radiation hazards (for both ionising and non-ionising radiation), and to provide information and advice to support protection from radiation hazards. During 1995, the Board published a formal statement[134] and the report of an Advisory Group[135] on the health effects of ultraviolet radiation, which strongly endorsed the Health of the Nation campaign[1] to reduce the year-on-year increase in the incidence of skin cancers, particularly melanomas.

United Kingdom Transplant Support Service Authority

The United Kingdom (UK) Transplant Support Service Authority was established in 1991 to facilitate the matching and allocation of organs for transplantation. It maintains the NHS organ donor register; by December, over 2.25 million people had registered their willingness to donate their organs in the event of sudden death.

Public Health Laboratory Service Board

The Public Health Laboratory Service provides microbiology and epidemiology services throughout England and Wales to protect the population from infection. A new strategic programme of re-organisation and service development started in 1995.

Microbiological Research Authority

The Centre for Applied Microbiology and Research at Porton Down continues to make a valuable contribution to public health research. Current projects relate to pathogenesis, diagnostics, therapeutics, vaccines and environmental microbiology.

National Creutzfeldt-Jakob Disease Surveillance Unit

This Unit was established in 1990, following the advent of bovine spongiform encephalopathy (BSE), to monitor any changes in the incidence or nature of the human illness, Creutzfeldt-Jakob disease.

Bioethics

Research ethics committees: Proposals for streamlining ethical approval of multi-centre studies were developed and good practice in local ethical review was promoted.

Bioethics in Europe: The Council of Europe's draft Bioethics Convention was considered.

Human genetics: The report of the House of Commons Select Committee on Science and Technology's inquiry into human genetics was published in July[136].

Human Fertilisation and Embryology Authority: A patient's guide to donor insemination and in-vitro fertilisation clinics was published[137], and advice given on extending the storage period for frozen embryos.

Gene Therapy Advisory Committee: The Gene Therapy Advisory Committee met three times in 1995, approved three gene therapy research protocols, and published a booklet which provides advice on writing information leaflets for patients who participate in gene therapy research[138].

Protection and use of patient information: The Department prepared guidance for the NHS on the protection and use of patient information.

Complaints

DH's plans for a new simplified complaints procedure for the NHS were published in March[139].

Research and development

The Department's R&D strategy promotes strong links with the science base, other major research funders in this country, and with EU research and technology programmes.

Use of information technology in clinical care

Development of the infrastructure needed to provide information to support clinical care continued, with progress in the electronic patient record, Read Code and decision support projects, introduction of the International Classification of Diseases version 10 (ICD-10) and new NHS numbers, and further support for training.

Dental health

Dental health of the nation: A dental survey as part of the Diet and Nutrition Survey of children aged $1^1/_2$ to $4^1/_2$ years was published in March[140].

General dental services: Proposals to improve NHS dentistry were announced in April after consultation on the Green Paper *Improving NHS dentistry*[141].

Community dental services: The community dental service retains responsibility for monitoring the dental health of the population and for dental health education and preventive programmes, and has wider responsibilities to patients who are unable or unwilling to obtain treatment from the general dental services.

Hospital dental services: The number of hospital dentists in England rose by 1.5% between September 1993 and September 1994. New outpatient referrals to consultant clinics fell by 1.5% in 1994/95 compared with 1993/94.

Continuing education and training for dentists: On 1 October, there were 517 trainees in 48 regionally based vocational training programmes.

Dental research: As well as dental aspects of the Diet and Nutrition Survey programmes, a co-ordinated NHS R&D programme for primary dental care was announced in June[142].

INTERNATIONAL HEALTH

England, Europe and health

The UK shares many health challenges with the rest of Europe, and the opportunity to work together on common problems brings substantial benefits. European programmes and initiatives allow countries to pool their experience and knowledge, and to take advantage of the greater resources that international co-operation brings into play.

The European Union: During 1995, the European Community (EC) continued its programme of public health initiatives. Final decisions were reached on proposals on AIDS and certain communicable diseases, cancer and health promotion. Formal adoption by the European Parliament and Council of Ministers of these programmes, and of a fourth programme on drug dependence, are expected in 1996. The European Commission also brought forward a proposal on health monitoring in October 1995; proposals on pollution-related illnesses, accidents and injuries, and rare diseases are expected during 1996. The Commission proposed that the High Level Committee on Health should be given formal status; the Committee considered issues such as future work on public health research and the integration of public health requirements across all Community policies. European Chief Medical Officers met to exchange views on the professional aspects of EC policies. The number of health professionals from Member States of the European Economic Area (EEA) working in the UK remains small, and most come for short periods to gain experience. EC Social Security Regulation 1408/71 continued to operate satisfactorily, co-ordinating health care cover for people moving between EEA Member States.

Council of Europe: During 1995, the Council of Europe continued its work on blood, organ transplantation, bioethics and the joint WHO/EC/Council of Europe European Network of Health Promoting Schools Project.

Relations with Central and Eastern Europe: By the end of 1995, eight Central and Eastern European countries had applied for membership of the EU. The Department continued to support exchange visits by specialists between the UK and countries in Central and Eastern Europe.

The Commonwealth

The theme of the 11th triennial Commonwealth Health Ministers' Meeting, held in Cape Town in December, was 'Women and health'. Health Ministers agreed recommendations for action by Governments and the Commonwealth Secretariat.

World Health Organization

European Regional Committee: At the 45th session of the Committee in September, Member States agreed on the need to give greater emphasis to the control of communicable diseases in the eastern part of the Region.

Executive Board: In January, the Board adopted a resolution urging the Director General to reallocate at least 5% of the programme budget to priority areas including communicable diseases, reproductive health, primary care and the environment.

World Health Assembly: In May, the World Health Assembly agreed a zero-rate-of-growth budget for the 1996-97 biennium, with a small increase to take account of global inflation and international currency fluctuations.

References

1. Department of Health. *The Health of the Nation: a strategy for health in England.* London: HMSO, 1992 (Cm. 1986).
2. Department of Health. *On the State of the Public Health: the annual report of the Chief Medical Officer of the Department of Health for the year 1992.* London: HMSO, 1993; 2.
3. Department of Health. *On the State of the Public Health: the annual report of the Chief Medical Officer of the Department of Health for the year 1993.* London: HMSO, 1994; 2.
4. Department of Health. *On the State of the Public Health: the annual report of the Chief Medical Officer of the Department of Health for the year 1994.* London: HMSO, 1995; 2.
5. Bone M, Bebbington A, Jagger C, Morgan K, Nicolaas G. *Health expectancy and its uses.* London: HMSO, 1995.
6. Will RG, Ironside JW, Zeidler M, et al. A new variant of Creutzfeldt-Jakob disease in the UK. *Lancet* 1996; **347:** 945-8.
7. Working Party on Bovine Spongiform Encephalopathy. *Report of the Working Party on Bovine Spongiform Encephalopathy.* London: Department of Health, 1989. Chair: Sir Richard Southwood.
8. Department of Health. *New variant of Creutzfeldt-Jakob Disease (CJD).* London: Department of Health, 1996 (Professional Letter: PL(CMO(96)5).
9. Department of Health. New variant of Creutzfeldt-Jakob Disease. *CMO's Update* 1996; **11**: 4-5.
10. Department of Health. *The Health of the Nation: briefing pack.* London: Department of Health, 1996.
11. Office of Population Censuses and Surveys. *General Household Survey 1994.* London: HMSO, 1996 (Series GHS no. 25).
12. Department of Health. *On the State of the Public Health: the annual report of the Chief Medical Officer of the Department of Health for the year 1991.* London: HMSO, 1992; 122-4.
13. Department of Health. *On the State of the Public Health: the annual report of the Chief Medical Officer of the Department of Health for the year 1992.* London: HMSO, 1993; 6, 122-3.
14. Department of Health. *On the State of the Public Health: the annual report of the Chief Medical Officer of the Department of Health for the year 1993.* London: HMSO, 1994; 2, 127-9.
15. Department of Health. *On the State of the Public Health: the annual report of the Chief Medical Officer of the Department of Health for the year 1994.* London: HMSO, 1995; 5-6, 144-5.
16. Department of Health. *Inpatients formally detained in hospitals under the Mental Health Act 1983 and other legislation: England: 1989-90 to 1994-95.* London: Department of Health, 1996 (Statistical Bulletin 1996/10).
17. *The Mental Health Act 1983.* London: HMSO, 1983.
18. Ritchie J. *Report of the Inquiry into the Care and Treatment of Christopher Clunis.* London: HMSO, 1994.
19. Blom-Cooper L, Hally H, Murphy E. *The falling shadow: one patient's mental healthcare 1978-1993.* London: Duckworth, 1995.
20. Department of Health, Home Office. *Review of health and social services for mentally disordered offenders and others requiring similar services: final summary report.* London: HMSO, 1992 (Cm. 2088).

21. Department of Health, Home Office. *Review of health and social services for mentally disordered offenders and others requiring similar services: volume 2: service needs: the reports of the community, hospital and prison advisory groups and an overview by the steering committee.* London: HMSO, 1993. Chair: Dr John Reed.

22.` Department of Health, Home Office. *Review of health and social services for mentally disordered offenders and others requiring similar services: volume 3: finance, staffing and training: the reports of the finance and staffing and training advisory groups.* London: HMSO, 1993. Chair: Dr John Reed.

23. Department of Health, Home Office. *Review of health and social services for mentally disordered offenders and others requiring similar services: volume 4: the academic and research base: the reports of the academic development and research advisory groups.* London: HMSO, 1993. Chair: Dr John Reed.

24. Department of Health, Home Office. *Review of health and social services for mentally disordered offenders and others requiring similar services: volume 5: special issues and differing needs: the report of the official working group on services for people with special needs.* London: HMSO, 1993. Chair: Dr John Reed.

25. Department of Health, Home Office. *Review of health and social services for mentally disordered offenders and others requiring similar services: volume 6: race, gender and equal opportunities.* London: HMSO, 1993. Chair: Dr John Reed.

26. Department of Health, Home Office. *Review of health and social services for mentally disordered offenders and others requiring similar services: volume 7: people with learning disabilities (mental handicap) or with autism.* London: HMSO, 1993. Chair: Dr John Reed.

27. Home Office. *Custody, care and justice: the way ahead for the prison service in England and Wales.* London: HMSO, 1991.

28. HM Prison Service Health Care Directorate. *Health care standards for prisons in England and Wales.* London: HM Prison Service, 1994.

29. Advisory Committee on the Microbiological Safety of Food. *Report on verocytotoxin-producing Escherichia coli.* London: HMSO, 1995.

30. Department of Health. *On the State of the Public Health: the annual report of the Chief Medical Officer of the Department of Health for the year 1993.* London: HMSO, 1994; 5, 74-112.

31. Department of Health. *On the State of the Public Health: the annual report of the Chief Medical Officer of the Department of Health for the year 1994.* London: HMSO, 1995; 7, 88-127.

32. Department of Health. *On the State of the Public Health: the annual report of the Chief Medical Officer of the Department of Health for the year 1994.* London: HMSO, 1995; 7-8.

33. Department of Health. *Variations in health: what can the Department of Health and the NHS do?* London: Department of Health, 1995.

34. NHS Executive. *Priorities and planning guidance: 1996/97.* Wetherby (West Yorkshire): Department of Health, 1995.

35. Advisory Committee on the Microbiological Safety of Food. *Report on poultry meat.* London: HMSO, 1996.

36. *The Food Safety (General Food Hygiene) Regulations 1995.* London: HMSO, 1995 (Statutory Instrument: SI 1995 no. 1763).

37. *The Food Safety (Temperature Control) Regulations 1995.* London: HMSO, 1995 (Statutory Instrument: SI 1995 no. 2200).

38. Lord President's Office. *Tackling drugs together: a strategy for England: 1995-1998.* London: HMSO, 1995 (Cm. 2846).

39. Health Education Authority. *A parents' guide to drugs and solvents.* London: Health Education Authority, 1995.

40. Department of Health, Task Force to Review Services for Drug Misusers. *Report of an independent review of drug treatment services in England.* London: Department of Health, 1996.

41. Taylor JC, Norman CL, Bland JM, Ramsey JD. *Trends in deaths associated with abuse of volatile substances: 1971-1994.* London: St George's Hospital Medical School, 1996 (report no. 9).

42. Committee on Safety of Medicines. *Combined oral contraceptives and thromboembolism.* London: Committee on Safety of Medicines, 1995.

43. Department of Health. Venous thromboembolism and oral contraceptives that contain desogestrel or gestodene. *CMO's Update* 1995; **8:** 2.

44. World Bank. *World Development Report 1995: investing in health.* New York: Oxford University Press, 1995.

45. Department of Health. *Health of the Nation key area handbook: mental illness, 2nd edn.* London. HMSO, 1994.

46. Jenkins R, Meltzer H. The National Survey of Psychiatric Morbidity in Great Britain. *Soc Psychiatry Psychiatr Epidemiol* 1995; **30:** 1-4.

47. Jenkins R. Towards a system of outcome indicators for mental health care. *Br J Psychiatry* 1990; **157:** 500-14.

48. Wing J, Curtis R, Beevor A. *HoNOS: Health of the Nation Outcome Scales.* London: Royal College of Psychiatrists, 1996.

49. Department of Health. *The spectrum of care: local services for people with mental health problems.* Wetherby (West Yorkshire): Department of Health, 1996.

50. Department of Health. *24-hour nursed care for people with severe and enduring mental illness.* Wetherby (West Yorkshire): Department of Health, 1996.

51. Boyce JM. Patterns of MRSA prevalence. *Infect Control Hospital Epidemiol* 1991; **12:** 78-82.

52. Noble WC. *Microbiology of human skin, 2nd edn.* London: Lloyd Luke Medical, 1981.

53. Emmerson AM, Enstone JE, Griffin M, Kelsey MC, Smyth ETM. The second national prevalence survey of infection in hospitals: overview of the results. *J Hosp Infect* 1996; **32:** 175-90.

54. Hospital Infection Society, British Society for Antimicrobial Chemotherapy. Revised guidelines for the control of epidemic methicillin-resistant *Staphylococcus aureus. J Hosp Infect* 1990; **16:** 351-77.

55. Department of Health. *Improving the effectiveness of the NHS.* London: Department of Health, 1994 (Executive Letter: EL(94)74).

56. Department of Health. *Methicillin resistant Staphylococcus aureus in community settings.* Wetherby (West Yorkshire): Department of Health, 1996 (Professional Letter: PL/CMO(96)3, PL/CNO(96)1, CI(96)12).

57. Department of Health, Public Health Laboratory Service. *Hospital infection control: guidance on the control of infection in hospitals.* London: Department of Health, 1995 (Health Service Guidelines: HSG(95)10).

58. Public Health Laboratory Service. Outbreak of hospital acquired multidrug resistant tuberculosis. *Commun Dis Rep* 1995; **5:** 161.

59. Public Health Laboratory Service. Multidrug resistant tuberculosis in a London hospital. *Commun Dis Rep* 1996; **6:** 205.

60. Department of Health. *Protection and use of patient information.* Wetherby (West Yorkshire): Department of Health, 1996 (Health Service Guidelines: HSG(96)18).

61. Office of Population Censuses and Surveys. *General Household Survey 1994.* London: HMSO, 1996 (Series GHS no. 25).

62. Office of Population Censuses and Surveys. *General Household Survey 1988.* London: HMSO, 1990 (Series GHS no. 19).

63. Office of Population Censuses and Surveys. *General Household Survey 1989.* London: HMSO, 1991 (Series GHS no. 20).

64. Gupta S. Health Surveys as a tool for government: the Health Survey for England as a paradigm case. *Arch Public Health* 1994; **52:** 99-113.

65. Bennett N, Dodd T, Flatley J, Freeth S, Bolling K. *Health Survey for England 1993.* London: HMSO, 1995.

66. Department of Health. *Sensible drinking: the report of an Inter-Departmental Working Group.* London: Department of Health, 1995.

67. Department of Health. *Nutrition guidelines for hospital catering.* London: Department of Health, 1995.

68. Department of Health. *Obesity: reversing the increasing problem of obesity in England: a report from the Nutrition and Physical Activity Task Forces.* London: Department of Health, 1995.

69. Gregory JR, Collins DL, Davies PSW, Hughes JM, Clarke PC. *National Diet and Nutrition Survey: children aged $1\frac{1}{2}$ to $4\frac{1}{2}$ years.* London: HMSO, 1995.

70. House of Commons Health Committee. *Inquiry into children's health.* London: House of Commons Health Committee, 1995 (Press Notice 1994/95-15).

71. *Reporting of Injuries, Diseases and Dangerous Occurrences Regulations (RIDDOR) 1995.* London: HMSO, 1995 (Statutory Instrument: SI 1995, no. 3163).

72. Office of Population Censuses and Surveys, Health and Safety Executive. *Occupational health: the Registrar General's decennial supplement for England and Wales*. London: HMSO, 1995 (Series DS no. 10).

73. Department of Health. *NHS responsibilities for meeting continuing health care needs*. Wetherby (West Yorkshire): Department of Health, 1995 (Health Service Guidelines: HSG(95)8, Local Authority Circular: LAC(95)5).

74. Department of Health. *Fit for the future: second progress report on the Health of the Nation*. London: Department of Health, 1995.

75. Meltzer H, Gill B, Petticrew M, Hinds K. *The prevalence of psychiatric morbidity among adults living in private households*. London: HMSO, 1995 (OPCS Surveys of Psychiatric Morbidity in Great Britain: report 1).

76. Meltzer H, Gill B, Petticrew M, Hinds K. *Physical complaints, service use and treatment of adults with psychiatric disorders*. London: HMSO, 1995 (OPCS Surveys of Psychiatric Morbidity in Great Britain: report 2).

77. Meltzer H, Gill B, Petticrew M, Hinds K. *Economic activity and social functioning of adults with psychiatric disorders*. London: HMSO, 1995 (OPCS Surveys of Psychiatric Morbidity in Great Britain: report 3).

78. Meltzer H, Gill B, Petticrew M, Hinds K. *The prevalence of psychiatric morbidity among adults living in institutions*. London: HMSO, 1996 (OPCS Surveys of Psychiatric Morbidity in Great Britain: report 4).

79. Meltzer H, Gill B, Petticrew M, Hinds K. *Physical complaints, service use and treatment of residents with psychiatric disorders*. London: HMSO, 1996 (OPCS Surveys of Psychiatric Morbidity in Great Britain: report 5).

80. Meltzer H, Gill B, Petticrew M, Hinds K. *The economic activity and social functioning of residents with psychiatric disorders*. London: HMSO, 1996 (OPCS Surveys of Psychiatric Morbidity in Great Britain: report 6).

81. Meltzer H, Gill B, Petticrew M, Hinds K. *Psychiatric morbidity among homeless people*. London: HMSO, 1996 (OPCS Surveys of Psychiatric Morbidity in Great Britain: report 7).

82. Foster K, Meltzer H, Gill B, Petticrew M, Hinds K. *Adults with a psychotic disorder: living in the community*. London: HMSO, 1996 (OPCS Surveys of Psychiatric Morbidity in Great Britain: report 8).

83. Sartorius N, Ustun T, Costa E Silva J. An international study of psychological problems in primary care: preliminary report from the WHO collaborative project on psychological problems in general health care. *Arch Gen Psychiatry* 1993; **50**: 819-24.

84. Goldberg D, Huxley P. *Common mental disorders: a biosocial model*. London: Routledge, 1992.

85. Department of Health. *Health and personal social services statistics for England*. London: HMSO, 1995.

86. Confidential Inquiry into Homicides and Suicides by Mentally Ill People. *A preliminary report on homicides*. London: Royal College of Psychiatrists, 1994.

87. Steering Committee of the Confidential Inquiry into Homicides and Suicides by Mentally Ill People. *Report of the Confidential Inquiry into Homicides and Suicides by Mentally Ill People*. London: Royal College of Psychiatrists, 1996.

88. Department of Health, Social Services Inspectorate, Department of Education. *A handbook on child and adolescent mental health*. London: HMSO, 1995.

89. Health Advisory Service. *Child and adolescent mental health services: together we stand: the commissioning role and management of child and adolescent mental health services*. London: HMSO, 1995.

90. Department of Health. *Caring for people: the care programme approach for people with a mental illness referred to the specialist psychiatric services*. London: Department of Health, 1990 (Health Circular: HC(90)23).

91. NHS Management Executive. *Introduction of supervision registers for mentally ill people from 1 April 1994*. Leeds: Department of Health, 1994 (Health Service Guidelines: HSG(94)5).

92. Department of Health and Social Security. *Better services for the mentally handicapped*. London: HMSO, 1980.

93. Social Services Inspectorate. *Leisure and recreation facilities*. London: Social Services Inspectorate, 1996.

94. *The NHS and Community Care Act 1990*. London: HMSO, 1990.

95. Paykel ES, Jenkins R. *Prevention in psychiatry: report of the Special Committee on the Place of Prevention in Psychiatry.* London: Gaskell, 1994.
96. Jenkins R, Griffiths S, Hawton K, Morgan G, Tylee A, Wylie I, eds. *The prevention of suicide.* London: HMSO, 1994.
97. Kingdon DG, Jenkins R. *Suicide prevention.* In: Phelan M, Thornicroft G, eds. *Emergency psychiatric services.* London: Routledge, 1995.
98. Jenkins R, Warman D. *Promoting mental health policies in the workplace.* London: HMSO, 1993.
99. Department of Health. *Caring for people: community care the next decade and beyond.* London: HMSO, 1989 (Cm. 849).
100. Department of Health. *The patient's charter.* London: Department of Health, 1991.
101. Research and Development Task Force. *Supporting research and development in the NHS.* London: HMSO, 1994. Chair: Professor Anthony Culyer.
102. House of Lords Select Committee on Science and Technology. *Medical research and the NHS reforms report: 1994-95 Session.* London: HMSO, 1995 (HL Paper 12).
103. Department of Health. *Government Response to the Third Report of the House of Lords Select Committee on Science and Technology: medical research and the NHS reforms: 1994-95 Session.* London: HMSO, 1995 (Cm. 2984).
104. Department of Health. *Public health in England: roles and responsibilities of the Department of Health and the NHS.* London: Department of Health, 1994.
105. Department of Health. *Making it happen: the contribution, role and development of nurses, midwives and health visitors: report of the Standing Nursing and Midwifery Advisory Committee.* Wetherby (West Yorkshire): Department of Health, 1995 (Executive Letter: EL(95)58).
106. National Confidential Enquiry into Peri-operative Deaths. *The Report of the National Confidential Enquiry into Peri-operative Deaths.* London: National Confidential Enquiry into Peri-operative Deaths, 1994.
107. National Advisory Body on the Confidential Enquiry. *Report of the Confidential Enquiry into Stillbirths and Deaths in Infancy (CESDI): 1 January-1 December.* London: Department of Health, 1995.
108. Department of Health, Welsh Office. *A policy framework for commissioning cancer services: a report by the Expert Advisory Group on Cancer to the Chief Medical Officers of England and Wales: guidance for purchasers and providers of cancer services.* London: Department of Health, 1995.
109. Department of Health. *Advisory Group on Osteoporosis: report.* London: Department of Health, 1994. Chair: Professor David Barlow.
110. Department of Health. *Strategic review of pathology services.* London: HMSO, 1995.
111. Office of Population Censuses and Surveys. *The OPCS monitoring scheme for congenital malformations: a review by a working group of the Registrar General's Medical Advisory Committee.* London: HMSO, 1995 (Occasional paper no. 43).
112. Department of Health, British Diabetic Association. *St Vincent Joint Task Force for Diabetes: the report: 1995.* London: Department of Health, 1995.
113. Thomas K, Fall M, Parry G, Nicholl J. *National survey of access to complementary health care via general practice.* Sheffield: Medical Care Research Unit, University of Sheffield, 1995.
114. HM Prison Service. *Drug misuse in prison.* London: HM Prison Service, 1995.
115. Public Health Laboratory Service. The incidence and prevalence of AIDS and prevalence of other severe HIV disease in England and Wales for 1995 to 1999: projections using data to the end of 1994: report of an Expert Group convened by the Director of the Public Health Laboratory Service on behalf of the Chief Medical Officers. *Commun Dis Rev* 1995; **6(1):** R1-R24.
116. Department of Health, Hospital Infection Working Group. *Hospital infection control: guidance on the control of infection in hospitals prepared by the Hospital Infection Working Group of the Department of Health and Public Health Laboratory Service.* Wetherby (West Yorkshire): Department of Health, 1995 (Health Service Guidelines: HSG(95)10).
117. Department of Health, Welsh Office, Scottish Office Home and Health Department, Northern Ireland Department of Health and Social Security, PHLS Communicable Disease Surveillance Centre. *Health information for overseas travel.* London: HMSO, 1995.
118. Department of Health, Committee on the Medical Effects of Air Pollutants. *Non-biological particles and health.* London: HMSO, 1995. Chair: Professor Stephen Holgate.

119. Department of Health, Committee on the Medical Effects of Air Pollutants. *Asthma and outdoor air pollution.* London: HMSO, 1995.

120. Department of Health, Advisory Group on the Medical Aspects of Air Pollution Episodes. *Health effects of exposures to mixtures of air pollutants: 4th report of the Advisory Group on the Medical Aspects of Air Pollution Episodes.* London: HMSO, 1995.

121. Committee on Medical Aspects of Radiation in the Environment, Radioactive Waste Management Advisory Committee. *Report on potential health effects and possible sources of radioactive particles found in the vicinity of the Dounreay nuclear establishment.* London: HMSO, 1995.

122. Ministry of Agriculture, Fisheries and Food. *Dioxins in food: 31st report of the Steering Group on Chemical Aspects of Food Surveillance.* London: HMSO, 1992; 46-9 (Food Surveillance Paper no. 31).

123. Ministry of Agriculture, Fisheries and Food. *Dioxins in food.* London: Ministry of Agriculture, Fisheries and Food, 1995 (Food Safety Information Bulletin no. 63).

124. Department of Health. *Carbaryl.* London: Department of Health, 1995 (Professional Letter: PL/CMO(95)4, PL/CNO(95)3).

125. Department of Health. Organophosphate sheep dips. *CMO's Update* 1995; **7**: 6.

126. Department of Health Medical Workforce Standing Advisory Committee. *Planning the medical workforce: second report.* London: Department of Health, 1995.

127. Department of Health. *Hospital doctors: training for the future: the report of the Working Group on Specialist Medical Training.* London: Department of Health, 1993. Chair: Dr Kenneth Calman.

128. *The European Specialist Medical Qualifications Order 1995.* London: HMSO, 1995 (Statutory Instrument: SI 1995 no. 3208).

129. *Health Authorities Act 1995.* London: HMSO, 1995.

130. *The Medical (Professional Performance) Act 1995.* London: HMSO, 1995.

131. Department of Health. *Maintaining medical excellence: review of guidance on doctors' performance: final report.* London: Department of Health, 1995.

132. NHS Executive. *Hospital locum doctors: the report of the Locums Working Group: a consultative document.* Leeds: Department of Health, 1995.

133. Department of Health. *The patient's charter: blood donors: interim charter.* London: Department of Health, 1995.

134. National Radiological Protection Board. *Board statement on effects of ultraviolet radiation on human health.* Oxford: National Radiological Protection Board, 1995 (Doc. NRPB 6, no. 2).

135. National Radiological Protection Board. *Health effects from ultraviolet radiation: report of an Advisory Group on Non-ionising Radiation.* Oxford: National Radiological Protection Board, 1995 (Doc. NRPB 6, no. 2).

136. House of Commons Select Committee on Science and Technology. *Human genetics: the science and its consequences.* London: HMSO, 1995.

137. Human Fertilisation and Embryology Authority. *The patients' guide to DI and IVF clinics.* London: Human Fertilisation and Embryology Authority, 1995.

138. Gene Therapy Advisory Committee. *Writing information leaflets for patients participating in gene therapy research.* London: Department of Health, 1995.

139. Department of Health. *Acting on complaints: the Government's proposals in response to 'Being heard', the report of a review committee on NHS complaints procedures.* Wetherby (West Yorkshire): Department of Health, 1995 (Executive Letter: EL(95)37).

140. Gregory JR, Collins DL, Davies PSW, Hughes JM, Clarke PC, Hinds K. *National Diet and Nutrition Survey: children aged $1^1/2$ to $4^1/2$ years: vol. 2: report of the dental survey.* London: HMSO, 1995.

141. Department of Health. *Improving NHS dentistry.* London: HMSO, 1994 (Cm. 2625).

142. Department of Health. *Dental specialisation will develop dentists' skills, says Gerald Malone.* London: Department of Health, 1995 (Press Release: H95/272).

Communications from the Chief Medical Officer to the medical profession and others during 1995

Copies of CMO letters and *CMO's Updates* can be obtained from: Department of Health Mailings, Two Ten Communications Ltd, Building 150 Thorp Arch Trading Estate, Wetherby, West Yorkshire LS23 7EH.

CMO Letters

Hepatitis C and blood transfusion look back (Professional Letter: PL/CMO(95)1) (3 April).
Influenza vaccine (Professional Letter: PL/CMO(95)2) (28 September).
Implementing the reforms to specialist medical training (Professional Letter: PL/CMO(95)3) (20 October).
Carbaryl (Professional Letter: PL/CMO(95)4, PL/CNO(95)3) (6 November).

CMO'S Update

CMO's Update 5 (March). Includes: Diphtheria immunisation and treatment; Unlinked anonymous HIV prevalence monitoring in England and Wales; Mental health in London Task Force Project; Direct referral to audiology clinics from general practice; Advisory Group on Medical Education, Training and Staffing; Changes in the regulations on epilepsy and driving; Nutritional aspects of cardiovascular disease; National surveys of psychiatric morbidity; NHS Health Survey Advice Centre.

CMO's Update 6 (July). Includes: Cancer services; Kawasaki disease; European Environment and Health Committee: Action Plan; Medical fitness to drive; Advisory Group on Medical and Dental Education, Training and Staffing (AGMETS); Silicone gel breast implants; Changes to specialist medical training; Influenza immunisation; Success of measles/rubella immunisation campaign; Health advice to travellers; Alert cards and information sheets for asplenic patients; Epidemiological overview of asthma; Child and adolescent mental health services; Sun exposure and skin cancer; Morbidity statistics from general practice 1991-1992; Finding beds for mentally disordered offenders; Health of the Nation and hospital doctors; Verocytotoxin-producing *Escherichia coli*.

CMO's Update 7 (October). Includes: On the State of the Public Health; Meningococcal infection; Strategic Review of Pathology Services; Schoolgirl rubella immunisation programme to be ended; Monovalent diphtheria vaccine for adults (low dose); Influenza vaccine; Workplace health promotion; Cervical spine instability in people with Down syndrome; Folic acid and the prevention of neural tube defects; Food-handlers: fitness to work; Shared care of drug misusers; Organophosphate sheep dips; New measures to reduce temazepam misuse.

CMO's Update 8 (November). Includes: Measles, rubella (MR) immunisation campaign 1994: one year on; Venous thromboembolism and oral contraceptives that contain desogestrel or gestodene; Advice to boil water to prevent cryptosporidiosis in immunocompromised patients; Guidelines on pregnancy loss and the death of a baby; Carbon monoxide; Carbaryl.

Public health Link

Copies of Public Health Link Communications can be obtained from: The Chief Medical Officer, Richmond House, 79 Whitehall, London SW1A 2NS.

Electronic cascade messages

Hepatitis C and blood transfusion (CEM/CMO(95)1) (11 January).
Measles immunisation (CEM/CMO(95)2) (28 April).
Ebola outbreak in Zaire (CEM/CMO(95)3) (18 May).
Combined oral contraceptives and thromboembolism (CEM/CMO(95)4) (19 October).
Carbaryl (CEM/CMO(95)5) (7th November).
Meningococcal infection: BBC TV Watchdog programme (CEM/CMO(95)6) (12 December).

CHAPTER 1

VITAL STATISTICS

(a)   Population size

The estimated resident population of England at 30 June 1995 was 48.9 million, an increase of some 196,000 (0.4%) compared with 1994. There was a natural increase (the excess of births over deaths) of approximately 96,000 and net inward migration and other changes of around 100,000 between mid-1994 and mid-1995.

(b)   Age and sex structure of the resident population

Appendix Table A.1 shows how the sizes of populations in various age-groups have changed in the period 1981-91 and in each of the subsequent years. The number of children below school age (0-4 years) has remained fairly stable in recent years, but shows a decrease between mid-1994 and mid-1995. The population of children of school age (5-15 years) continues to increase slowly, after falling during the 1980s. The relatively small late-1970s birth cohorts are now entering the youngest working age-group (16-29 years), the size of which is consequently declining. Larger cohorts born in the period after World War II, up to and including the 1960s, are now in the older working age-groups (30-64 years for men and 30-59 years for women); these groups are increasing in size. Numbers in the youngest pensioner age-group (65-74 years for men and 60-74 years for women) remain fairly stable. Up to 1994, those aged 75-84 years have fallen slightly in number as survivors from the small cohorts born during World War I reached this age-group; however, there was an increase in this age-group between mid-1994 and mid-1995, as those born in the peak year of 1920 have entered this age-group. The most elderly group (aged 85 years and over) continues to increase rapidly and represents a growing proportion of all pensioners. Just under two-thirds of persons above pensionable age (65 years for men and 60 years for women), and about three-quarters of those aged 85 years and over, are women.

(c)   Fertility statistics - aspects of relevance for health care

Total conceptions

Data on conceptions relate to pregnancies which led to a maternity or to a legal termination under the Abortion Act 1967[1,2]; they exclude spontaneous and illegal abortions. The latest available data relate to 1993 when 776,800 conceptions occurred to women resident in England, a fall of 1% from 1992 (see Table 1.1). The overall conception rate in 1993 was 76.3 per 1,000 women aged 15-44 years.

Total live births

Table 1.2 shows that there were 613,257 live births in England in 1995, 2.5% fewer than in 1994. This was the fifth successive decrease in annual births.

Table 1.1: *Conceptions by outcome, England, 1988, 1992 and 1993*

Age of woman	1988	1992	1993
Under 16 *			
Number (000s)	8.2	6.8	6.8
Rate			
Total	9.4	8.4	8.0
Maternities	4.3	4.1	3.8
Abortions	5.0	4.3	4.2
Under 20 †			
Number (000s)	113.3	87.3	81.3
Rate			
Total	66.4	61.4	59.3
Maternities	42.3	40.0	38.4
Abortions	24.1	21.4	20.9
All ages ‡			
Number (000s)	804.6	784.9	776.8
Rate			
Total	77.3	76.4	76.3
Maternities	61.9	61.5	61.5
Abortions	15.4	14.9	14.7

* Rates per 1,000 females aged 13-15 years.

† Rates per 1,000 females aged 15-19 years.

‡ Rates per 1,000 females aged 15-44 years.

Source: OPCS/ONS

Table 1.2: *Live births and proportion of live births outside marriage, crude birth rate, general and total period fertility rates, and sex ratio, England, 1985, 1994 and 1995*

Year of birth	Live births	Crude birth rate*	General fertility rate†	Total period fertility rate (TPFR)	Percentage of live births outside marriage	Sex ratio
1985	619301	13.1	60.9	1.78	19.5	105.4
1994	628956	13.0	61.9	1.74	32.2	105.6
1995	613257	12.6‡	60.4‡	1.70‡	33.7	105.1

* Births per 1,000 population of all ages.

† Births per 1,000 females aged 15-44 years.

‡ Provisional (based on 1994 population figures).

Note: Sex ratio represents number of male births per 100 female births.

Source: OPCS/ONS

The total period fertility rate (TPFR) measures the average number of children that would be born per woman if current age-specific fertility rates continued throughout her childbearing years. The TPFR in England was 1.70 in 1995, compared with 1.74 in 1994. The latest figure is only slightly above the lowest recorded level of 1.66 in 1977. The TPFR for England has now remained below 2.1, the level which would give long-term 'natural' replacement of the population, since 1972.

The proportion of live births occurring outside marriage has continued to increase slowly, reaching 33.7% of all births in 1995. Over half of these births were jointly registered by parents who were living at the same address, and presumably cohabiting.

Fertility of women aged 40 years and over

Although total fertility is declining slowly, the trend over recent years to delay childbearing has led to some increases in the age-specific fertility rates for older women. These have occurred for women aged 30-39 years, but they have been most pronounced for women aged 40-44 years, among whom there was a 28% increase in the fertility rate between 1990 and 1995 (see Table 1.3). Older

Table 1.3: *Numbers and rates of live births to women aged 40 years and over, England, 1990, 1994 and 1995*

Woman's age (years)	Numbers of births		
	1990	1994	1995
40	3636	3976	4287
41	2313	2692	2828
42	1506	1581	1692
43	917	954	967
44	435	537	536
40-44	*8807*	*9740*	*10310*
45	205	222	246
46	96	107	119
47	52	47	56
48	38	25	30
49	26	18	19
45-49	*417*	*419*	*470*
50 and over	58	49	37
40 and over	9282	10208	10817
Rates per 1,000			
40-44	5.08	6.12	6.48[*]
45-49	0.34	0.27	0.30[*]

[*] Provisional (based on 1994 population figures).

Source: OPCS/ONS

Table 1.4: *Maternities with multiple births by age of mother, England and Wales, 1985 and 1995*

Age of mother (years)	1985			1995		
	Total	Twins only	Triplets and over	Total	Twins only	Triplets and over
Numbers						
All ages	6803	6700	103	9038	8749	289
Under 20	320	320	-	291	289	2
20-24	1677	1660	17	1306	1288	18
25-29	2375	2341	34	2906	2821	85
30-34	1628	1591	37	2993	2871	122
35-39	707	694	13	1348	1293	55
40 and over	96	94	2	194	187	7
Rates per 1,000 maternities						
All ages	10.4	10.3	0.2	14.1	13.6	0.4
Under 20	5.6	5.6	-	6.9	6.9	0.1
20-24	8.7	8.6	0.1	10.0	9.9	0.1
25-29	10.5	10.4	0.2	13.5	13.1	0.4
30-34	13.0	12.7	0.3	16.7	16.0	0.7
35-39	16.1	15.8	0.3	20.9	20.0	0.9
40 and over	12.9	12.6	0.3	17.3	16.6	0.6

Note: Rates for women aged under 20 years and aged 40 years and over are based upon the population of women aged 15-19 and 40-44 years, respectively; total rates may not match sum of twins/triplets and over due to rounding.

Source: OPCS/ONS

women also have higher (and faster growing) rates of multiple maternities than do women at the younger fertile ages. In 1995, women aged 40 years and over had 17 multiple maternities per 1,000 total maternities, compared with 21 per 1,000 for women aged 35-39 years, but only 10 per 1,000 for women aged 20-24 years (see Table 1.4).

Conceptions to girls aged under 16 years

In 1993, there were 8.0 conceptions per 1,000 girls aged 13-15 years in England as a whole, compared with 8.4 per 1,000 in 1992 and 9.3 per 1,000 in 1991. Rates quoted for individual District Health Authorities (DHAs) have been calculated for the three years 1991-93, combined together to smooth erratic annual figures based upon very small numbers of events. Table 1.5 shows the highest and lowest conception rates per 1,000 girls aged 13-15 years over the three years, ranging from 16.5 in Barnsley to 3.4 in South West Surrey for total conceptions. Manchester had the highest rate for conceptions leading to maternities, and Doncaster and Barnsley had the highest rates for conceptions terminated by legal abortions per 1,000 girls aged under 16 years.

Table 1.5: *Districts with highest and lowest conception rates among girls aged under 16 years, England, 1991-93*

Area of usual residence	Rates per 1,000 girls aged 13-15 years		
	Total*	Maternities	Abortions
Areas with high rates			
Barnsley	16.5	7.8	8.7
Doncaster	15.8	7.1	8.8
Manchester	15.6	10.6	5.0
South-East London	15.1	7.8	7.2
Sandwell	14.7	8.2	6.5
Areas with low rates			
South West Surrey	3.4	1.2	2.2
Barnet	4.1	1.9	2.2
Huntingdon	4.1	1.6	2.5
East Surrey	4.3	2.0	2.3
Mid Surrey	4.4	1.4	2.9
Kingston and Richmond	4.4	1.6	2.8

*Totals may not match separate maternities and abortions figures due to rounding.

Source: OPCS/ONS

Abortions

A total of 149,764 abortions were performed in 1994 under the Abortion Act 1967[1,2] for women who were resident in England. This represents a decrease of 1,158 (0.8%) compared with 1993, but an increase of 19,613 (15%) compared with 1984. Of the total, 89% were carried out at under 13 weeks gestation, and only 3% were performed beyond 16 weeks gestation.

In 1994, 29% of all abortions carried out on resident women were for those aged 20-24 years; 13% were for those aged 35 years and over. The abortion rate was highest among women aged 20-24 years (25.6 abortions per 1,000 women aged 20-24 years).

In 1994, 18% of legal abortions were performed on women aged under 20 years; of these, 11% were for girls aged under 16 years. A comparison of abortion rates among those aged under 20 years for the years 1984 and 1994 showed no change in the rate of 16.2 abortions per 1,000 women aged 14-19 years.

References

1. *Abortion Act 1967.* London: HMSO, 1967.
2. *Abortion Act 1967 (as amended by Statutory Instrument: SI 480c.10).* London: HMSO, 1991.

(d)   Mortality

There were 529,038 deaths registered in England in 1995, a 2.2% increase compared with the 517,614 deaths in 1994, but fewer than the 541,121 deaths registered in 1993. The crude mortality rate fell from 11.1 per 1,000 population in 1993 to 10.6 per 1,000 in 1994, and then rose to a provisional rate (based on mid-1994 population estimates) of 10.9 per 1,000 in 1995.

1993 and 1994 mortality data

As reported last year[1], the Office for National Statistics (ONS, formed by the amalgamation of the Office of Population Censuses and Surveys (OPCS) and the Central Statistical Office) recently carried out an extensive redevelopment of its collection and processing system for mortality data. This process included the progressive computerisation of registration in local offices; the move to a large deaths database to hold all deaths data from 1993; and the introduction of automated coding of cause of death. As a result of the changes to the way in which deaths are coded, and other changes which occurred during 1993 (such as the temporary withdrawal of medical inquiries for obtaining additional details from certifying doctors on cause of death), 1993 and subsequent years' mortality data for some causes of death are not directly comparable with those for 1992 and earlier years.

Mortality rates 1985-95

Figures 1.1 and 1.2 show that over the decade 1985-95, mortality rates for males and females alike fell for most age-groups. However, the mortality rate for men aged 15-44 years rose by 7.5% between 1985 and 1990. This then fell between 1990 and 1993, but has since risen to be 5% higher in 1995 than in 1985. The downward trend in mortality rates among those aged 75 years and over stopped in 1992, and there may even be slight signs of an upturn in the rates. Mortality rates among children aged 1-14 years have fallen dramatically since 1988 - by 31% among boys and 25% among girls. The 1995 rates in the figures are provisional as they are based on 1994 population estimates.

Reference

1. Department of Health. *On the State of the Public Health: the annual report of the Chief Medical Officer of the Department of Health for the year 1994.* London: HMSO, 1995; 46.

(e)   Prevalence of disease in the community

Prevalence of treated disease

In 1994, the OPCS/ONS took over the management of the General Practice Research Database (formerly the VAMP Research Databank). Over 400 general practices in England and Wales contribute anonymised clinical and therapy data on nearly 3 million patients. These have been used to estimate the 1994 prevalence rates of disease diagnosed and treated by general practitioners (GPs).

Figure 1.1: *Percentage change in age-specific mortality rates, males,*
England, 1985-95 (1985=100)

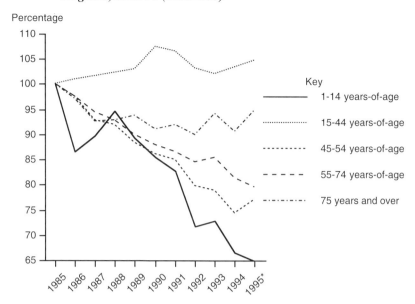

*Provisional data based on 1994 population estimates.

Source: OPCS/ONS

Figure 1.2: *Percentage change in age-specific mortality rates, females,*
England, 1985-95 (1985=100)

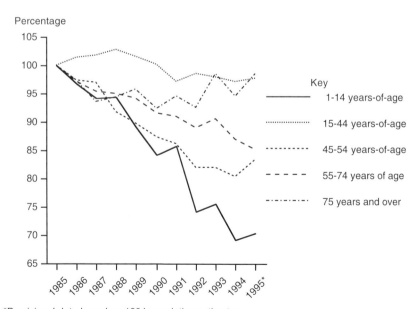

*Provisional data based on 1994 population estimates.

Source: OPCS/ONS

Asthma

In 1994, 6.4% of the population were prescribed asthma drugs, and had a diagnosis of asthma. In children aged 5-15 years, treated asthma was more common among boys: over 12% of boys received medication during the year (see Figure 1.3) compared with less than 10% of girls. In the 16-74 years age-group, asthma was more common among women. The data show a rise in treated asthma after 55 years, particularly among men. Some of this increase may be because there is an overlap in the way that doctors diagnose asthma and chronic obstructive airways disease. Two-thirds of people with treated asthma had been treated with corticosteroids.

Depression

In 1994, 9.8% of women and 4.1% of men aged 16 years and over in England and Wales had had a diagnosis of depression recorded at some time and had been prescribed antidepressants during the course of the year (see Figure 1.4). Treatment rates increased steeply with age and were roughly twice as high for women as for men in all age-groups. For women, treated depression was highest in the northern Regional Health Authorities (Northern, North Western, Mersey) and lowest in the Thames regions and Oxford (see Figure 1.5).

Figure 1.3: *Prevalence of treated asthma by age, males and females, England and Wales, 1994*

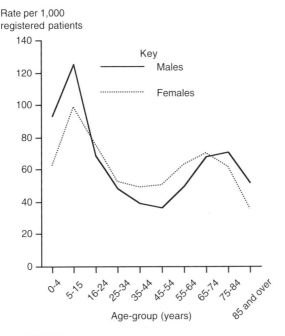

Source: OPCS/ONS

54

Figure 1.4: *Prevalence of treated depression by age, males and females, England and Wales, 1994*

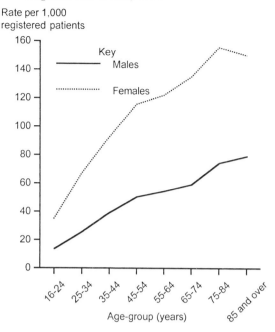

Source: OPCS/ONS

Figure 1.5: *Prevalence of treated depression by Region, females aged 16 years and over, England, 1994*

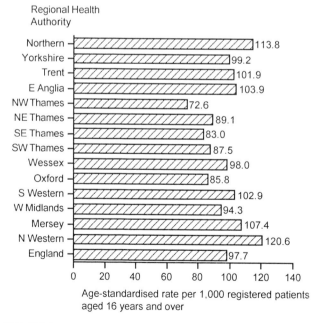

Source: OPCS/ONS

Figure 1.6: *Prevalence of treated hypertension by age, males and females, England and Wales, 1994*

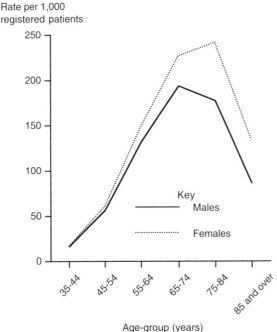

Source: OPCS/ONS

Hypertension

In 1994, 11.7% of women and 9.2% of men aged 35 years and over had a diagnosis of hypertension, and had been treated with antihypertensive drugs during the year; the proportion treated generally increased with age, although rates dropped in the very oldest age-groups (see Figure 1.6).

Chronic sickness

The General Household Survey (GHS)[1] is a continuous survey collecting information about 18,000 adults and 5,000 children in Great Britain each year. It provides two measures of self-reported chronic sickness. Firstly, people are asked whether they have any long-standing illness, disability or infirmity. Those who answer yes are then asked "What is the matter with you?", and then whether this limits their activities in any way. Acute sickness is measured by asking whether, in the two weeks before interview, people had to cut down on any of the things they usually do because of illness or injury. In 1994, 32% reported a long-standing illness, 19% a limiting long-standing illness and 14% restricted activity in the previous two weeks. Figure 1.7 shows trends from 1979 to 1994 for these three measures for males and females separately. The data are presented as three-year moving averages to smooth out year-on-year fluctuations. The prevalence of acute sickness has changed little. The prevalence of reported long-standing illness increased during the 1980s; towards the end of the decade the increase slowed, and then a slight fall occurred.

Figure 1.7: *Three-year moving averages of measures of morbidity from the General Household Survey, males and females, Great Britain, 1979-94*

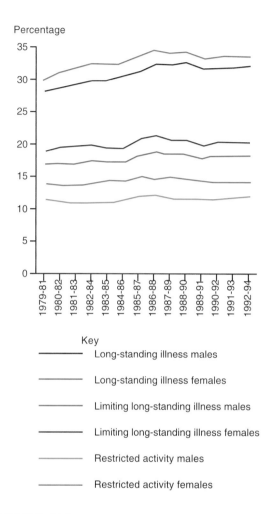

Key

——————— Long-standing illness males

——————— Long-standing illness females

——————— Limiting long-standing illness males

——————— Limiting long-standing illness females

——————— Restricted activity males

——————— Restricted activity females

Source: OPCS/ONS, GHS

Limiting long-term illness data from the 1991 Census

A question on long-term illness was also asked in the 1991 Census. The proportions of the population with a limiting long-term illness appears to vary among different ethnic groups, even when age-standardised to allow for different age structures[2]. Men and women of Bangladeshi and Pakistani origin reported the highest age-standardised rates, and those of Chinese ethnic groups the lowest. Traditional industrial areas also tended to have high age-standardised rates.

Health Survey data

The type of condition reported as the cause of long-standing illness was analysed by International Classification of Diseases (ICD) group in the 1989 and 1994[1] GHS, and also in the 1991, 1993 and 1994 Health Surveys for England[3,4,5]. Illnesses associated with the musculo-skeletal system were most frequently mentioned as the cause of long-standing illness, followed by the heart and circulatory system and the respiratory system.

References

1. Office of Population Censuses and Surveys. *General Household Survey 1994*. London: HMSO, 1996 (Series GHS no. 25) (in press).
2. Charlton J, Wallace M, White I. Long-term illness: results from the 1991 Census. *Population Trends* 1994; **75**.
3. Office of Population Censuses and Surveys. *Health Survey for England 1991*. London: HMSO, 1993 (Series HS no. 1).
4. Office of Population Censuses and Surveys. *Health Survey for England 1993*. London: HMSO, 1995 (Series HS no. 3).
5. Social and Community Planning Research. *Health Survey for England 1994*. London: HMSO (in press).

(f) Infant and perinatal mortality

Provisional statistics for 1995 in England indicate that there were 3,721 infant deaths (babies who died under one year-of-age) compared with 3,861 in 1994. Of this total, 2,545 (68%) died in the neonatal period (under 28 days-of-age), and 1,176 (32%) in the post-neonatal period (between 28 days and one year-of-age). The infant mortality rate remained constant between 1994 and 1995 at 6.1 per 1,000 live births, the lowest rate ever recorded (see Appendix Table A.5).

Based on provisional statistics, during 1995 in England there were 3,406 stillbirths compared with 3,584 in 1994. Thus the stillbirth rate fell between 1994 and 1995 from 5.7 to 5.5 per 1,000 total births (live births and stillbirths). One-quarter of these stillbirths were recorded as babies who died between 24 and 27 weeks gestation. (On 1 October 1992, the legal definition of a stillbirth was altered from a baby born dead after 28 complete weeks gestation or more to one born dead after 24 complete weeks gestation or more; comparisons with earlier years must take this change in legal definition into account.) The perinatal mortality rate (stillbirths and deaths of babies under 7 days-of-age per 1,000 total births) fell marginally from 8.9 in 1994 to 8.8 in 1995.

Appendix Table A.5 also shows that the post-neonatal mortality rate in England has fallen consistently every year since 1988. Between 1988 and 1995, it fell by over 50% from 4.1 to 1.9 per 1,000 live births. Most of this fall can be accounted for by a 71% reduction in the post-neonatal sudden infant death mortality rate (with a mention on the death certificate of 'cot death', sudden infant death syndrome [SIDS], or a similar term) over the period 1988 to 1994. The highest annual fall in post-neonatal sudden infant deaths occurred between 1991 and 1992; between 1993 and 1994, the post-neonatal sudden infant death mortality rate in England remained unchanged at 0.6 per 1,000 live births.

Figure 1.8: *Infant mortality by father's occupational status, England, 1983-94*

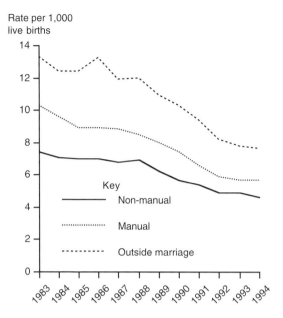

Source: OPCS/ONS

Figure 1.8 shows infant mortality rates by the father's occupation (for births within marriage) for the period 1983-94. Babies of fathers in non-manual occupations had consistently lower mortality rates than babies of fathers in manual occupations.

(g)   Trends in cancer* incidence and mortality

Data from the 1988 and 1989 GHS[1,2] show that 1% of adults reported cancer as a cause of long-standing illness. This estimate can be compared with that based on the OPCS/ONS Longitudinal Study (LS), which is discussed in the report of the 1990 review of the cancer registration system[3]. The LS brings together, for 1% of the population, information from the National Cancer Registration Scheme, successive Censuses and death registrations. It indicates that just over half a million people alive in 1981 would have had a cancer registered in the preceding ten years - again a prevalence of around 1%.

The latest totals of cancer registrations for England and Wales relate to 1991. Appendix Tables A.7 and A.8 show the provisional numbers registered by age, sex and site; these are based on semi-aggregated data supplied by the regional cancer registries to OPCS/ONS. Although trends over the period 1979-91 must be interpreted with caution, for all malignant neoplasms (excluding non-

---

* cancer = malignant neoplasm

melanoma skin cancer) there were increases of about 10% for males and 20% for females. When specific sites of malignancy are examined there are some trends of note.

When adjusted for age, lung cancer registration decreased for males but increased for females between 1979 and 1991. For both sexes there were large increases in the number of registrations of malignant melanoma of the skin during the period 1979-91. During the same period the long-term decline in registrations of stomach cancer continued. There were marked downward trends for lymphosarcoma and reticulosarcoma and for Hodgkin's disease, but an upward trend for other malignant neoplasms of lymphoid and histiocytic tissue, to which less well-specified lymphomas would be coded.

There have been upward trends for cancers of the prostate, and kidney and other unspecified urinary organs between 1979 and 1991. As a result of a change in coding practice, the number of registrations of carcinoma-in-situ of the cervix uteri was very much higher in 1984 than in previous years. The number fell between 1990 and 1991 by 5% - but, in 1991, the total number of registrations was over four times that in 1979; possible improvements in the level of completeness of registration and in ascertainment need to be taken into account.

As with the incidence of all cancers, there has been no decline in mortality in recent years. Age-standardised death rates since the 1920s are shown in the 1992 Report[4]. For males, the post-war rise levelled off in the 1970s. For females, there was a declining trend until the early 1960s, followed by a rise. Within these totals, however, there was a rise and then a fall in the rate for cancer of the lung/bronchus in males, contrasting with a rise in females. There was a steady fall in the rate for cancer of the stomach in both sexes. There has been a sharp decline in mortality from breast cancer since 1990.

References

1. Office of Population Censuses and Surveys. *General Household Survey 1988*. London: HMSO, 1990 (Series GHS no. 19).
2. Office of Population Censuses and Surveys. *General Household Survey 1989*. London: HMSO, 1991 (Series GHS no. 20).
3. Office of Population Censuses and Surveys. *Review of the national cancer registration system: report of the Working Group of the Registrar General's Medical Advisory Committee*. London: HMSO, 1990 (Series MB1 no. 17).
4. Department of Health. *On the State of the Public Health: the annual report of the Chief Medical Officer of the Department of Health for the year 1992*. London: HMSO, 1993; 44.

(h)   Trends in reporting congenital anomalies

Appendix Table A.6 shows the number of babies notified who had selected congenital anomalies. The provisional 1995 rate in England decreased to 80.7 per 10,000 live births, 1% lower than in 1994 and 28% lower than in 1990. The rate for stillbirths decreased to 2.7 per 10,000 total births, 10% lower than in 1990.

An exclusion list was introduced in January 1990 to identify minor anomalies which should no longer be notified. As a result, the total number of notifications received fell by 4,058 (34%) between 1989 and 1990. This fall was accounted for entirely by a decrease in notifications of live births with anomalies. Three groups shown in the table were affected by the exclusion list: ear and eye malformations, cardiovascular malformations and talipes. For these three groups the comments in the following paragraphs are restricted to the changes that took place between 1990 and 1995; for the remainder, the comments refer to the changes between 1985 and 1995.

Since 1985, there has been a reduction in the rate of central nervous system anomalies for live births (from 8.9 to 2.8 per 10,000 live births) and stillbirths (from 1.8 to 0.8 per 10,000 total births). Conditions such as hydrocephalus and anencephaly, which are within the group most likely to be detected prenatally by diagnostic ultrasound or alphafetoprotein screening, have shown the largest fall. A similar decrease has been reported in other countries.

The rate of hypospadias/epispadias has approximately halved since 1980; in 1995 the rate was 7.5 per 10,000 live births. Since 1990, the rate of ear and eye anomalies per 10,000 live births has fallen from 5.7 to 3.0, and that of talipes from 14.9 to 10.5. For cardiovascular anomalies, the rate per 10,000 live births has decreased from 6.8 to 6.2.

CHAPTER 2

THE NATION'S HEALTH

(a)   Recent health trends in England

Life expectancy at birth in England in 1994 reached an estimated 74.5 years for males and 79.7 years for females. Striking improvements in life expectancy have occurred over recent years, although occasional small reductions have been observed - as may be the case in 1995 when estimated from the latest data. However, average life expectancy has improved substantially over the last 25 years, by over 5 years for men and 4 years for women.

The overall level of health in a population must not be judged by trends in mortality alone. Nevertheless, such trends supplement the wide range of morbidity and health-related behaviour data presented elsewhere in this Report, aid identification of certain major health problems and enable progress to be assessed.

Over the 25 years from 1970 to 1995, the overall mortality rate - all causes adjusted for age differences - has fallen by 30%, reflecting substantial reductions in every age-group from birth to 85 years and over. The fall was slightly greater among men (32%) than women (29%). The decline in the mortality rate among those aged under 65 years has, allowing for differences in age structure, fallen more steeply over this period, by 39% - the fall again being greater among men (42%) than for women (37%). Particularly large falls in mortality have occurred among young children, with reductions exceeding 60% seen in the 1-4 and 5-9 years age-groups.

The major causes of death are illustrated in Figure 2.1. The predominant causes of death are circulatory diseases and cancers, which together account for over two-thirds of all deaths. The mortality rate for circulatory diseases has fallen by 43% between 1970 and 1995; the major constituents of this category, coronary heart disease (CHD) and stroke, have both shown sizeable falls since 1970 - CHD mortality rates falling by 32% and stroke mortality by over 50%. Again, the reduction in mortality rates among people aged under 65 years was more marked over this period, with falls of 47% for CHD and 58% for stroke.

The main components of cancer mortality are shown in Figure 2.2. Although the overall mortality rate for cancers (all causes combined, adjusted for age differences) was apparently little different in the early 1990s from that of 20 years earlier, this tends to obscure some important changes which have occurred in recent years. The overall cancer mortality rate, adjusted for age differences, altered little between 1970 and the early to mid-1980s. Since then, mortality rates have fallen by about 7% (10% in men, 4% in women). If deaths under the age of 65 years are considered, mortality rates in males have been falling

Figure 2.1: *Major causes of death, all ages, males and females, England and Wales, 1995*

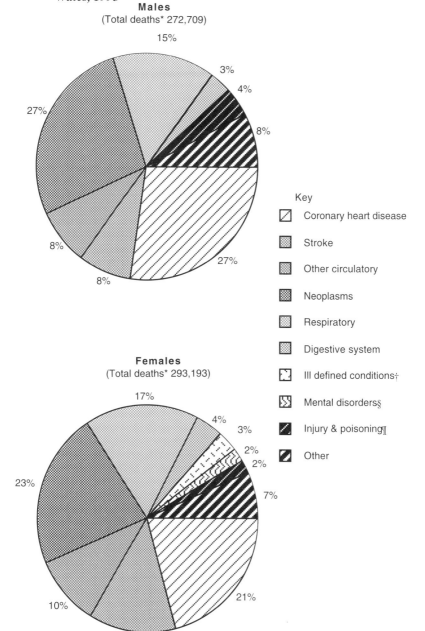

Males
(Total deaths* 272,709)

15%
3%
4%
8%
27%
27%
8%
8%
8%

Key

⬜ Coronary heart disease

⬜ Stroke

⬜ Other circulatory

⬜ Neoplasms

⬜ Respiratory

⬜ Digestive system

⬜ Ill defined conditions†

⬜ Mental disorders§

⬛ Injury & poisoning¶

⬛ Other

Females
(Total deaths* 293,193)

17%
4%
3%
2%
2%
7%
23%
21%
10%
13%

*Figures for individual cause categories exclude deaths at under 28 days-of-age; numbers may not total 100% because of rounding.
†Includes 'senility'.
§Includes dementia.
¶Includes suicides and accidents.

Source: CHMU from OPCS/ONS data

Figure 2.2: *Main causes of cancer deaths, all ages, males and females, England and Wales, 1995*

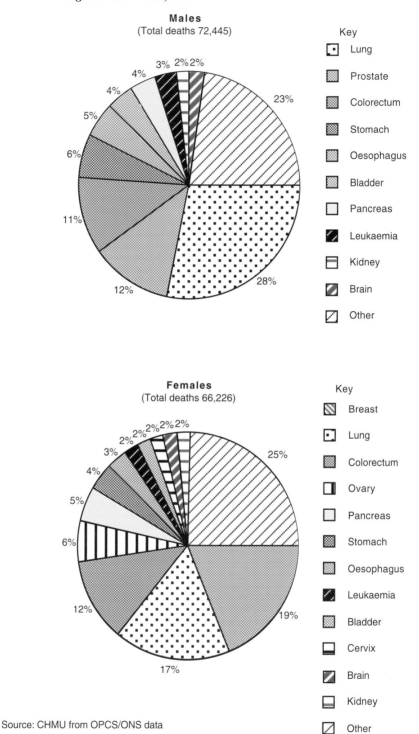

Source: CHMU from OPCS/ONS data

throughout the 25-year period (down 30%), whilst among women mortality rates were static between 1970 and the early 1980s, since when they have declined by more than 15%. Major contributors to the recent reduction in cancer mortality among women aged under 65 years are falls in breast cancer (mortality down by almost 15% since 1989), and lung cancer which has fallen by around 20% since 1988. However, lung cancer mortality among women aged over 70 years continues to rise.

These trends are generally encouraging but must be set against international data. For example comparison with other European Union (EU) countries indicates that this country continues to have relatively high mortality rates for both CHD and cancers. Nevertheless the trends among younger adults, particularly in the most recent years, are encouraging.

Basic sources of information

Complementary to mortality data are statistics on morbidity. Some of these are from routine sources (eg, data on hospital admissions or GP consultations), but health surveys are also an essential component to monitoring of the health of the population because they can cover individuals who are not in contact with health care services, and they can collect data in a standardised fashion. Ideally such a survey should be national in scope, representative of the population from which it is drawn, comprehensive in its coverage of the topics on which it focuses, repeated at intervals to allow time trends to be assessed, and sufficiently large to permit comparisons across place and person.

The Health Survey for England comes very close to meeting all of these criteria[1]. This national survey covers a representative sample of the population living in private households, and from 1991-94 it focused on the prevalence of cardiovascular disease, its main risk factors, and the uptake of relevant services. It is repeated with a fresh sample annually and, since 1993, the Survey has had a greater sample size which makes it possible to provide prevalence estimates at regional level. The report of the 1993 Health Survey for England was published early in 1995[2], accompanied by a popular summary which was distributed widely and was well received. The report of the 1994 Survey will be published early in 1996.

In 1995, the Survey focus moved temporarily to new topics (asthma, accidents, disability) in addition to a core of items which will be repeated annually (eg socio-demographic variables, height and weight, and blood pressure). Also, for the first time, children aged 2-15 years were included. The 1996 Survey will cover asthma, accidents and special measures of general health in addition to the core topics. The 1997 Survey is likely to focus on children and young people in line with the Health of the Young Nation initiative, though the core items will continue to be included for a sample of adults as well.

The Health Survey for England is part of a wider Departmental health survey programme which includes, for example, the National Survey of Psychiatric Morbidity (see page 96) and the Dietary and Nutritional Surveys (see page 70).

References

1. Gupta S. Health Surveys as a tool for government: the Health Survey for England as a paradigm case. *Arch Public Health* 1994; **52**: 99-113.
2. Bennett N, Dodd T, Flatley J, Freeth S, Bolling K. *Health Survey for England 1993*. London: HMSO, 1995.

(b)   Inter-Departmental Group on Public Health

The Inter-Departmental Group on Public Health, chaired by the Chief Medical Officer, facilitates inter-Departmental discussion and exchange of information on health issues. The Group usually meets three times a year to keep under review hazards to public health; to provide advice to Government on the assessment of such hazards; to provide an inter-Departmental forum for the discussion of scientific or technical issues that bear on public health; and to strengthen and support existing links between the Department of Health (DH) and other Government Departments, and to identify and correct any gaps in communication. The composition of the Group reflects the public health interests of Government Departments.

(c)   Variations in health

Last year's Report[1] drew attention to the way in which variations in health are associated with gender, social class, geography, ethnicity and occupation. Such variations have been observed for more than a century.

However, while socio-economic, gender, regional and ethnic differences are widespread and are seen in all countries, the magnitude of these differences is not fixed; differences are recorded within and between countries and over different time periods, indicating that some variations at least are susceptible to change through intervention.

In 1994, the Chief Medical Officer set up a Working Group to report on how DH and the National Health Service (NHS) could tackle variations in health in the Health of the Nation key areas[2], and on what further research was needed. The Group's report[3] was published in October 1995, and was widely distributed to health and local authorities and others (see page 89).

The Working Group found that considerable activity was taking place within the NHS to try to tackle variations in health, but that much of this work was at the margins of health authority activity and little of it was being evaluated. A study commissioned from the Centre for Reviews and Dissemination (CRD) at York University to indicate what interventions had been shown to be effective found that the available evidence on effectiveness was very limited, and that there is a pressing need for more, and more rigorous, evaluation of interventions[4].

The report's main recommendations were that:

— health authorities and general practitioner purchasers should have a plan to identify and tackle variations and to evaluate interventions;

— such plans should include provision for working in alliance with other relevant bodies;

— health authorities, GP purchasers and NHS Trusts should monitor access to services to safeguard equitable access;

— DH should work actively in alliance with other Government Departments and other bodies to encourage social policies which promote health, hold the NHS to account for implementation of the recommendations that apply to the NHS, and take forward the report's recommendations on research;

— health authority purchasers should rigorously evaluate interventions which they implement;

— health authority purchasers should be supported in this task of evaluation by the establishment of a clearing house;

— the Medical Research Council (MRC), the Economic and Social Research Council and DH should co-ordinate their programmes of research; *and*

— a DH research consultation exercise should recommend priorities for the evaluation of interventions to address health variations, research to address the needs of particularly vulnerable groups of the population and basic research into causal processes.

A £2.4 million research initiative will be launched in 1996, drawing on the outcome of a research consultation exercise recommended by the Working Group and completed during 1995.

References

1. Department of Health. *On the State of the Public Health: the annual report of the Chief Medical Officer of the Department of Health for the year 1994.* London: HMSO, 1995; 64-5.
2. Department of Health. *The Health of the Nation: a strategy for health in England.* London: HMSO, 1992 (Cm. 1986).
3. Department of Health. *Variations in health: what can the Department of Health and the NHS do?* London: Department of Health, 1995.
4. NHS Centre for Reviews and Dissemination, University of York. *Review of the research on the effectiveness of health service interventions to reduce variations in health.* York: NHS Centre for Reviews and Dissemination, University of York, 1995.

(d)   Housing and health

The impact of housing on the environment and health has long been recognised. Despite improvements to the housing stock, there remains a need to reduce still further the level of unfit housing - particularly in respect of coldness and damp. Damp air in homes can have indirect effects on health, with particular risk of respiratory disease, and other aspects of indoor air quality also play a role. Poor maintenance of heating devices, especially gas fires and paraffin stoves, may lead to an accumulation of carbon monoxide in poorly ventilated rooms, and exposure to pollutants generated by gas cookers and open fires can cause adverse effects. However, environmental tobacco smoke remains the most important component of indoor air pollution. On the other hand, improvements in housing standards such as double glazing (which reduces ventilation), fitted carpets and central heating may encourage the multiplication of house dust mites, and exacerbate asthma.

Housing conditions can contribute to ill-health, but the relations between housing and health cannot be viewed only in terms of the physical quality of individual dwellings. Other inter-related factors include occupants' lifestyle, the local environment and access to adequate health and social services. These complex interactions mean that it is often difficult to establish or quantify links between housing and health, or to assess the possible impact of changing any one factor.

(e)   Substance misuse

In December, the report of an Inter-Departmental Group to review scientific and medical evidence on the health effects of drinking alcohol was published[1]. The report concluded that:

— moderate alcohol consumption confers some health benefits, mainly by giving protection against coronary heart disease (CHD) to men aged over 40 years and post-menopausal women. The maximum health advantage can be obtained from drinking between one and two units of alcohol daily;

— regular daily consumption of between three and four units for men, and between two and three units for women, will not cause significant health risk, with the exceptions noted below, but consistently drinking four or more units daily for men or three or more for women is not recommended because of the progressive health risk;

— pregnant women, and those trying to become pregnant, should not drink more than one or two units once or twice a week;

— more attention should be paid to the short-term effects of drinking alcohol, especially the need to avoid intoxication and to avoid alcohol consumption altogether in some circumstances, including driving; *and*

— parents and carers of children should ensure that children are aware of the hazards of alcohol and only consume it, if at all, in moderate quantities, having regard to their age and physical development.

The Health Education Authority (HEA) was awarded a contract to develop a health promotion campaign based on these messages in 1996.

In May, the Government launched its three-year anti-drugs strategy 'Tackling Drugs Together', focusing on crime, young people and the protection of public health[2].

The 1994 Home Office Addicts Index, published in July[3], showed that the number of notified drug addicts in the United Kingdom (UK) rose 21% to 33,952 (compared with 27,976 in 1993). DH also collects wider information on drug misuse, which is not directly comparable with that of the Home Office. Two *Drug Misuse Statistics Bulletins* were published for the 12 months to 30 September 1994[4,5]. The number of individual drug misusers in England presenting to services for the first time, or after an absence of six months or more, rose 7% to over 37,000 in that period.

The Task Force set up to review the effectiveness of services for drug misusers continued its work. An 18-month study is tracking over 1,100 drug misusers, and DH also funded eight pilot schemes to test the benefits of prescribing oral methadone within a structured maintenance programme. During the year, the Department provided an extra £1 million to fund 40 projects in 1995/96 to develop early intervention services for young people at risk or in the early stages of substance misuse.

The Department launched the National Drugs Helpline in April, providing a free, 24-hours-a-day service to give advice and information to drug misusers, their families and friends, and anyone else who requires information. The effectiveness of this service will be fully evaluated. DH also awarded a contract to the HEA to manage the drugs and solvents publicity budget for the three years of the *Tackling drugs together* strategy from April. The HEA launched a publicity campaign in November to promote awareness of the National Drugs Helpline. The campaign used advertising in the youth press and on independent radio and focused on the health risks associated with ecstasy (methylenedioxymethamphetamine or MDMA) misuse.

In June, St George's Hospital Medical School published the latest mortality data associated with volatile substance abuse. The number of deaths in 1993 was 75, a fall from the 84 reported for 1992[6]; 1994 figures indicate a further fall to 57. In April, the Advisory Council on the Misuse of Drugs published its report on volatile substance abuse[7]; DH is co-ordinating the Government's response to its recommendations.

References

1. Department of Health. *Sensible drinking: the report of an Inter-Departmental Working Group.* London: Department of Health, 1995.
2. Lord President's Office. *Tackling drugs together: a strategy for England: 1995-1998.* London: HMSO, 1995 (Cm. 2846).
3. Home Office. *Statistics of drug addicts notified to the Home Office, United Kingdom, 1994.* London: Home Office 1995 (Statistical Bulletin 95/17).

4. Department of Health. *Drug misuse statistics*. London: Department of Health, 1995 (Statistical Bulletin 95/8).
5. Department of Health. *Drug misuse statistics*. London: Department of Health, 1995 (Statistical Bulletin 95/24).
6. Taylor JC, Norman CL, Bland JM, Anderson HR, Ramsey JD. *Trends in deaths associated with abuse of volatile substances: 1971-1993*. London: Department of Public Health Services, St George's Hospital Medical School, 1994 (Report no.7).
7. Advisory Council on the Misuse of Drugs. *Volatile substance abuse*. London: HMSO, 1995.

(f)   Nutrition

In September, the Nutrition Task Force (NTF) launched *Nutrition guidelines for hospital catering*[1], which is being used by the NHS Executive to help to develop performance measures. In October, the NTF held its final meeting; it compiled a report for Ministers on progress, incorporating the outcomes of several specific projects and setting out recommendations for further progress.

Also in September, the NTF and the Physical Activity Task Force published their report *Obesity: reversing the increasing problem of obesity in England*[2]. This report recommended an increase in physical activity and a reduction in dietary fat as the two key aspects for prevention of obesity, and also suggested concentration of effort on at-risk groups. A systematic review of effective interventions for the prevention and treatment of obesity was commissioned (see page 81).

The Committee on Medical Aspects of Food and Nutrition Policy (COMA; known before 1995 as the Committee on Medical Aspects of Food Policy) set up a working group to prepare guidelines for Government, industry and professionals on the nutritional assessment of modifications to infant milk formulas. A working group was also set up to review the dietary intakes and nutritional status of the population with regard to folic acid and the nutrients currently statutorily added to flour and yellow fats, particularly iron, calcium and vitamin D; and to consider mechanisms, including fortification of foods, for the maintenance of adequate nutritional status for these substances and for evaluation of their safety and effectiveness.

The report of the Diet and Nutrition Survey of children aged $1^1/_2$ to $4^1/_2$ years, part of the National Diet and Nutrition Survey (NDNS) programme, was published in March[3]. Field work for the NDNS survey of people aged 65 years and over was completed in October. Data collection for a survey of infant feeding among members of Asian communities continued throughout 1995, and a year of field work for the latest quinquennial survey of infant feeding practices started in September.

References

1. Department of Health. *Nutrition guidelines for hospital catering*. London: Department of Health, 1995.
2. Department of Health. *Obesity: reversing the increasing problem of obesity in England: a report from the Nutrition and Physical Activity Task Forces*. London: Department of Health, 1995.
3. Gregory JR, Collins DL, Davies PSW, Hughes JM, Clarke PC. *National Diet and Nutrition Survey: children aged $1^1/_2$ to $4^1/_2$ years*. London: HMSO, 1995.

(g)   Health of children

Survival prospects for children have continued to improve. Infant mortality remained at 6.1 per 1,000 live births in 1995 in England and Wales, the lowest recorded level. The mortality rate for children aged 1-19 years was 24 per 100,000.

Better understanding of the particular health needs of children and a fuller recognition of the lasting consequences of those factors that influence health and health-related behaviour in children led to the launch, in July, of the Health of the Young Nation initiative within the Health of the Nation strategy[1]. This initiative provides a focus on young people's health, and aims to ensure that they are equipped to make responsible and informed choices about their health and lifestyle.

In March, the NHS Executive issued a draft consultation document, *Child health in the community: a guide to good practice*[2]. There was a keen response with many valuable comments. The final guidance will complement an earlier document, *Welfare of children and young people in hospital*[3], and is intended to assist those in the NHS, local authorities and voluntary bodies who have responsibilities for purchasing and providing health services for children outside hospital.

The report of the Health of the Nation Variations Sub-Group, published in October[4], encompassed the implications for children's health of variations between socio-economic groups, different ethnic groups, and geographical variations. The recommendations of the Sub-Group will guide further action to understand the origins of such variations, with a view to developing strategies to reduce them (see page 89).

In July, the Parliamentary Health Select Committee announced that it would conduct an inquiry into children's health[5]. The deliberations of the Committee will stimulate further consideration of the factors, including service provision, which influence the health of children. The Committee is expected to report in 1996.

References

1. Department of Health. *The Health of the Nation: a strategy for health in England.* London: HMSO, 1992 (Cm. 1986).
2. Department of Health. *Child health in the community: a guide to good practice.* London: Department of Health, 1995.
3. Department of Health. *Welfare of children and young people in hospital.* London: HMSO, 1991.
4. Department of Health. *Variations in health: what can the Department of Health and the NHS do?* London: Department of Health, 1995.
5. House of Commons Health Committee. *Inquiry into children's health.* London: House of Commons Health Committee, 1995 (Press Notice 1994/95-15).

(h)   Health of adolescents

The Report for 1993[1] included a special chapter on the health of adolescents. There has since been increasing interest in the special health needs of young people, including the development of the Health of the Young Nation initiative (see page 79). The Parliamentary Health Select Committee announced in 1995 that it would consider the specific health needs of adolescents as part of its inquiry into children's health[2], which will take place in 1996 (see page 71).

In July, the NHS Executive's Central Research and Development Committee published the report of its multidisciplinary advisory group on priorities for NHS research in maternal and child health[3]. The report's priorities included issues relating to injury; disability; chronic disease; mental health; and promotion of healthy behaviours in children and adolescents, and such research is being co-ordinated by the Executive's South Thames Regional Office.

Much of the activity to promote the health of young people occurs in schools. DH and the Department for Education and Employment (DfEE) are funding the HEA to co-ordinate the European Network of Health Promoting Schools within the UK. The first report from this project (which was launched by the World Health Organization's Regional Office for Europe, the Commission of the European Community and the Council of Europe) was published in October[4]. As part of the Government's strategy *Tackling drugs together*[5] (see page 68), the DfEE published a circular on drug prevention and schools in May[6]. This was accompanied by curriculum guidance for schools[7] and a digest of drug education resources for schools[8].

DH funded two conferences on adolescent care in practice, organised by the Royal College of General Practitioners. The first of these was held in London in October, and a further conference will be held in Hull during 1996.

References

1. Department of Health. *On the State of the Public Health: the annual report of the Chief Medical Officer of the Department of Health for the year 1993.* London: HMSO, 1994; 5, 74-112.
2. House of Commons Health Committee. *Inquiry into children's health.* London: House of Commons Health Committee, 1995 (Press Notice 1994/95-15)
3. Department of Health. *Improving the health of mothers and children: NHS priorities for research and development: report to the NHS Central Research and Development Committee.* Leeds: Department of Health, 1995.
4. Health Education Authority, National Foundation for Educational Research in England and Wales. *The health promoting school: baseline survey.* London: Health Education Authority, 1995.
5. Lord President's Office. *Tackling drugs together: a consultation document on a strategy for England: 1995-1998.* London: HMSO, 1994 (Cm. 2678).
6. Department for Education and Employment. *Drug prevention and schools.* London: Department for Education and Employment, 1995 (DfEE Circular 4/95).
7. Department for Education and Employment, Schools Curriculum and Assessment Authority. *Drug education: curriculum guidance for schools.* London: Schools Curriculum and Assessment Authority, 1995.
8. Department for Education and Employment. *Digest of drug education resources for schools.* London: Department for Education and Employment, 1995.

(i)   Health of women

Women's health was highlighted in September at the Fourth United Nations (UN) World Conference on Women in Beijing, China (see page 228). A key commitment made by the UK Government during the conference was to "mainstream a gender perspective into all policies and programmes". The objective is to ensure that the needs of women and men alike are automatically considered as part of policy appraisal and service delivery. The development of gender-disaggregated statistics is integral to this process and district-level data of this kind appears in the public health common data set[1]; these data help Directors of Public Health (DsPH) to monitor the health of local populations, and should play a major role in monitoring performance against Health of the Nation targets[2], and give local planners, purchasers and providers of health care a powerful tool to compare health differences between men and women and for planning health promotion activity and other NHS services accordingly (see also below on men's health and page 89 on health variations). The aim is to ensure that where men and women have differing health needs, local services can set out to meet them. Although women in general live longer than men, they have specific health and health education needs - including those related to CHD, cancers, mental illness, sexual health, accidents, the menopause and osteoporosis.

At the close of the UN conference, a UK implementation plan was announced for the global platform for action, consulting and involving non-Governmental organisations as part of the process. Baroness Cumberlege, Parliamentary Under Secretary of State for Health in the House of Lords, who has responsibility for women's health issues, regularly meets the Women's Health and Screening Delegation for discussions; this Delegation is made up of representatives from 15 national women's organisations.

References

1. Department of Health, University of Surrey Institute of Public Health. *Health of the Nation: public health common data set 1994.* Guildford: Institute of Public Health, University of Surrey, 1995.
2. Department of Health. *The Health of the Nation: a strategy for health in England.* London: HMSO, 1992 (Cm. 1986).

(j)   Health of men

Men's survival has improved substantially over the past decade: average male life expectancy at birth in 1994 is estimated to be 74.5 years (projected to rise to 75.7 years by the year 2002), compared with 72.0 years in 1984. Nevertheless, these figures remain lower than the equivalents for women.

The key areas identified in the Health of the Nation initiative[1] have a major impact on men's health. Work carried out within the strategy during 1995 should help to improve men's health, and gender variations were featured in the report of the Variations Sub-Group of the Chief Medical Officer's Health of the Nation Working Group[2] (see page 89).

The workplace provides a helpful setting for informing men about health promotion messages. The work of the Health of the Nation Workplace Taskforce and the Workplace Health Advisory Team will be important in this area. As part of Europe Against Cancer (EAC) Week in October, a videotape was produced to disseminate the EAC code in workplaces.

Men's health was also the focus of initiatives outside the Department, following its emphasis in the 1992 Report[3]. For example, the Royal College of Nursing commissioned a survey of DsPH on this subject[4]; the research will inform the work of its men's health group. DH also funded a two-year research project by Community Health UK to ensure that health messages to men reach the intended audience.

To support the 1995 EAC week, the HEA published a report on cancers in men[5]. This generated further interest in and awareness of men's cancers and attitudes to health issues. A leaflet on testicular cancer was launched by the Hon Tom Sackville MP, the then Parliamentary Under Secretary of State for Health in the House of Commons, at a major international conference, 'Men's health matters', held in London in July; it has been distributed widely to universities, colleges and GPs[6]. Reports of research commissioned to consider the cost-effectiveness and clinical benefits of methods to detect and treat prostate cancer are expected in mid-1996.

References

1. Department of Health. *The Health of the Nation: a strategy for health in England.* London: HMSO, 1992 (Cm. 1986).
2. Department of Health. *Variations in health: what can the Department of Health and the NHS do?* London: Department of Health, 1995.
3. Department of Health. *On the State of the Public Health: the annual report of the Chief Medical Officer of the Department of Health for the year 1992.* London: HMSO, 1993; 6, 79-106.
4. Market and Opinion Research International (MORI). *Men's health: a survey of district directors of public health.* London: MORI, 1995.
5. Health Education Authority. *Report on men's cancers project.* London: Health Education Authority, 1995.
6. Department of Health. *A whole new ball game.* London: Department of Health, 1995.

(k)   Health of black and ethnic minorities

The Department is committed to improving the health of and access to health services for people from black and ethnic minorities, and the Report for 1991[1] drew attention to some of the differences in health and disease patterns seen among people from such communities.

To improve information about the health of ethnic minorities, DH funded further work on the analysis of ethnic data in the 1991 Census. This examination of the relations between ethnicity and health status, allowing for demographic, socio-economic and area factors, will start to become available in 1996.

A directory of ethnic minority initiatives, also funded by the Department, will be published during 1996, with details of all projects undertaken since 1988 by voluntary organisations and health authorities to improve both health and access to health services for ethnic minorities. The directory will be a valuable reference guide for health authorities and ethnic minority groups.

The Health of the Nation[2] key areas are all important for ethnic minority health, and DH has funded a number of relevant projects. For example, the Department funded a Cancer Research Campaign (CRC) conference in May to identify the health needs of ethnic minorities in relation to cancer. The conference brought together health professionals to review existing information and to set an agenda for further research.

Initiatives to support purchasers of health care continue. The King's Fund Centre was commissioned by DH to produce a tool-kit for improving services for people from black and ethnic minority communities, which will contain practical advice for purchasers and providers of health care to ensure that appropriate and culturally sensitive services are provided.

The NHS Ethnic Health Unit (EHU) continued to fund projects in the NHS to improve access to health care and to ensure that the views of local minority groups are taken into account in the commissioning and provision of such care. In its third year, the EHU will focus on good practice and clinical effectiveness in the primary care of people from ethnic minorities.

The NHS Executive continued to monitor and support implementation of the programme of action for NHS staff from ethnic minorities. Ethnic monitoring data on the entire NHS workforce have been collected and will be published early in 1996.

References

1. Department of Health. *On the State of the Public Health: the annual report of the Chief Medical Officer of the Department of Health for the year 1991.* London: HMSO, 1992; 8-9, 54-77.
2. Department of Health. *The Health of the Nation: a strategy for health in England.* London: HMSO, 1992 (Cm. 1986).

(l)   Health in the workplace

The special chapter on health in the workplace in last year's Report[1] set out the background to the development of occupational health practice in the UK, described the main occupational health hazards and illnesses, and identified some future developments. It emphasised the importance of risk assessment and management and pointed to the role that occupational health professionals can play to improve health at work.

The new Reporting of Injuries, Diseases and Dangerous Occurrences Regulations (RIDDOR) 1995[2], due to come into force on 1 April 1996, will extend and update the number of reportable diseases. The new list will include a range of additional work-related musculo-skeletal disorders, cancers, infections and occupational dermatitis. Explanatory information for GPs and other health professionals will be published in April 1996.

A study was established in 1995 to examine the feasibility of extending the existing voluntary reporting schemes (covering lung and skin disease) by the medical profession to provide information on musculo-skeletal disorders, hearing loss and other prominent work-related conditions. GPs may be the first point of contact for many occupationally related illnesses, and ways in which training can be incorporated into GP postgraduate education continue to be explored. In partnership with the Faculty of Occupational Medicine, the Health and Safety Executive (HSE) has planned a series of seminars on occupational health for GPs and is developing a complementary training package. As well as recognising work-related ill-health in patients, GPs also have to address risks to themselves and the staff whom they employ.

During 1995, progress with the HSE's Health Risk Review action programme continued. To expand the information base on the extent of ill-health caused by work, screening questions were included in the 1995 Labour Force Survey[3] to identify individuals who had suffered a work-related illness. Follow-up interviews and further information from medical practitioners were obtained where consent had been given. Results from these inquiries will add to existing knowledge about ill-health at work, and help in setting priorities and targets for future preventive and information programmes. One example of action on a specific risk is a revised programme for work-related upper limb disorders to improve understanding of their prevalence and severity, increase awareness of these conditions and encourage compliance with good practice by employers.

The HSE and the Office of Population Censuses and Surveys (OPCS), in collaboration with independent experts, published the *Occupational Health Decennial Supplement*, a major compendium of statistics of occupational health in England and Wales[4]. In May, the HSE launched its occupational health campaign, 'Good health is good business', which aims to raise awareness of occupational health risks, explain the value of preventive action and improve managerial competence in dealing with health issues[5]. Guidance includes indications for seeking specialist help from suitably trained occupational health professionals. A multi-agency group has been convened by DH to increase employers' awareness of mental health issues. A range of initiatives should encourage better co-ordination of work and also encourage improved ways of dealing with problems (see page 124).

Other HSE publications during the year included a booklet for employers providing advice on the nature and causes of work-related stress[6]; practical examples of how companies have controlled musculo-skeletal and noise hazards[7]; and guidance for employers and health practitioners on health surveillance in noisy industries[8,9].

Extensive research into employer practice in the provision of health surveillance at work has indicated some misunderstandings about its scope and application. HSE is to review its guidance in the light of the survey findings.

A study, jointly funded by the HSE, the Ministry of Agriculture, Fisheries and Food and DH has been set up to assess whether prolonged, low-level exposure to organophosphate sheep dips leads to chronic ill-health (see page 190). The Health and Safety Commission's Health Services Advisory Committee, in consultation with DH, produced a 10-year plan to improve health and safety performance across the health care sector[10].

During the year, the Advisory Committee on Dangerous Pathogens published guidance on protection against blood-borne infection in the workplace[11] and on the categorisation of biological agents[12]. Further guidance is likely to be issued during 1996 on infections in pregnancy; on the management of infection risks when working with experimental animals; and on the management of viral haemorrhagic fevers. Other research projects commissioned by the HSE during the year included manual handling and postures, and work-related stress.

The workplace is identified in the Health of the Nation White Paper[13] as one of the settings in which health promotion could most profitably be focused (see page 92). Over the last year, the Workplace Steering Group, a sub-group of the Wider Health Working Group, chaired by Baroness Cumberlege, Parliamentary Under Secretary of State for Health in the House of Lords, has taken forward recommendations of the Workplace Task Force to develop a practical action plan for workplace health promotion. The Steering Group's work has resulted in the production of the *ABC of health promotion in the workplace*[14]. Targeted at small and medium-sized companies, this information pack sets out the case for workplace health promotion, the scope for it to deliver benefits to businesses and to individuals, and provides details of organisations and publications as possible sources of help. The Steering Group also recommended setting up a small team to develop alliances between businesses, and other interested parties, to allow for more effective delivery of workplace health promotion.

References

1. Department of Health. *On the State of the Public Health: the annual report of the Chief Medical Officer of the Department of Health for the year 1994.* London: HMSO, 1995; 7, 88-127.
2. *Reporting of Injuries, Diseases and Dangerous Occurrences Regulations (RIDDOR) 1995.* London: HMSO, 1995 (Statutory Instrument: SI 1995, no. 3163).
3. Office of Population Censuses and Surveys. *Labour Force Survey 1995.* London: HMSO (in press).
4. Office of Population Censuses and Surveys, Health and Safety Executive. *Occupational health: the Registrar General's decennial supplement for England and Wales.* London: HMSO, 1995 (Series DS no. 10).
5. Health and Safety Executive. *Health risk management: a practical guide for managers in small and medium size enterprises.* London: Health and Safety Executive, 1995.
6. Health and Safety Executive. *Stress at work: a guide for employers.* London: Health and Safety Executive, 1995.
7. Health and Safety Executive. *Sound solutions: techniques to reduce noise at work.* London: Health and Safety Executive, 1995.
8. Health and Safety Executive. *Health surveillance in noisy industries: advice for employers.* London: Health and Safety Executive, 1995.
9. Health and Safety Executive. *A guide to audiometric testing programmes.* London: Health and Safety Executive, 1995.
10. Health Services Advisory Committee. *Management of health and safety in the Health Service.* London: Health and Safety Executive, 1991.
11. Advisory Committee on Dangerous Pathogens. *Protection against blood-borne infections in the workplace: HIV and hepatitis.* London: HMSO, 1995.

12. Advisory Committee on Dangerous Pathogens. *Categorisation of biological agents according to hazard and categories of containment.* Sudbury, Suffolk: Health and Safety Executive, 1995.
13. Department of Health. *The Health of the Nation: a strategy for health in England.* London: HMSO, 1992 (Cm. 1986).
14. Department of Health. *ABC of health promotion in the workplace: a resource pack for employers.* London: Department of Health, 1995.

(m)   Health of people in later life

The Department continues to promote services for older people to facilitate their independent life in the community. Further improvements in community health services and falling lengths of hospital stay have been mirrored by the growth of local authority provision in domiciliary services predominantly used by older people. In reviewing its priorities for the NHS, DH has placed emphasis on the need for sensitive hospital discharge practices, and high quality community and rehabilitation services. Particular priority has been given to the need for individual assessment, early detection of problems, and the development of more integrated patterns of service for older people through joint working between all relevant agencies.

DH continued to promote work on sickness and disability prevention for older people, which included research on health expectancy measures published in October[1]. An expert working group has been set up to look further at available measures of health state and possible future developments in data collection. DH has also supported the development of health mentoring projects and other initiatives using older volunteers, and of advice to GPs on health promotion for older people.

Guidance on NHS responsibilities for meeting continuing health care needs was issued in February[2]; this guidance confirmed and clarified the NHS's responsibilities for meeting a range of continuing health care needs, many of which will be found among elderly people. It aimed to achieve greater consistency across the country in the NHS provision of continuing health care, by setting out a national framework of criteria by which people will be eligible for such care. The guidance also included provision for panels which may review individual decisions about eligibility for NHS continuing inpatient care.

Health authorities have consulted with local authorities and other parties with an interest on their draft policies and criteria for continuing health care, and final versions should be put into operation on 1 April 1996.

References

1. Bone MR, Bebbington AC, Jagger C, Morgan K, Nicolaas G. *Health expectancy and its uses.* London: HMSO, 1995.
2. Department of Health. *NHS responsibilities for meeting continuing health care needs.* Wetherby (West Yorkshire): Department of Health, 1995 (Health Service Guidelines: HSG(95)8, Local Authority Circular: LAC(95)5).

CHAPTER 3

THE STRATEGY FOR HEALTH

(a)   Introduction

The Government's strategy for health in England was launched in July 1992 in the *Health of the Nation* White Paper[1]. This innovative initiative to improve the health of the entire population focused on five key areas responsible for much of the avoidable ill-health and premature death in England, and set out to redress the balance between health care (the treatment of ill-health) and health promotion - the preservation of good health and the development of better health.

The strategy recognised explicitly for the first time that health was not the exclusive preserve of the National Health Service (NHS) and the Department of Health (DH): a wide range of Government Departments' policies may affect health; an enormous range of organisations have the potential to influence health; and responsibility for health rests at all levels, including with the individual. The strategy identified a series of settings in which health promotion could profitably be targeted. It also developed the concept of health alliances, where joint working could get messages across to sectors of the population who might otherwise be hard to reach, and where partnerships could achieve more through working together than their members could individually.

In July, *Fit for the future: second progress report on the Health of the Nation*[2] was published. It showed encouraging progress towards most of the targets, but also areas where trends were in the wrong direction and work needed to be concentrated: the 1994 target for teenage smoking had not been reached; obesity was more common among men and women alike; and lung cancer incidence in women was not falling as rapidly as required. *Fit for the future*[2] also contained welcome news to show how widely the strategy now influences the work of the various partners identified in the White Paper[1]. December saw the publication of *Policy appraisal and health*[3] - guidance for other Government Departments and organisations such as local authorities which describes how to ensure that health implications can be taken into account during the development of any new policies.

During 1995, the Government strategy for health developed a new focus, the Health of the Young Nation; this followed interest generated by the special chapter on the health of adolescents in the 1993 Report[4]. The Health of the Young Nation initiative was launched jointly by Ministers from the Departments of Health, Education and Employment, and Transport at a conference held in July to mark the third anniversary of the strategy for health. This new initiative complements work specific to the five key areas of the strategy for health by taking a broader look at the health of young people and identifying influences on behaviours which are relevant across the key areas. DH identified the study of health-related behaviours, and how they might be changed, as a specific research area with a programme of research to be funded over five years. An initial review of existing work on health-related behaviours and effective health promotion has been commissioned. Promotion of healthy behaviours in young people was also among the priorities identified in 1995 by the NHS Executive's Central Research and Development Committee[5] (see page 72); and the Health Education Authority (HEA) is supporting research to identify young people's views on health issues and the effectiveness of different methods of health promotion.

Development of the Health of the Young Nation initiative relies on promoting health through a wide variety of agencies. DH has held meetings in 1995 with the representatives of the major faith communities within England, and with journalists providing advice to young people through teenage magazines. In October, the Department published a report[6] of two conferences which looked at the contribution that nurses, midwives and health visitors might make to achieving Health of the Nation targets as they relate to young people. In November, DH advertised for tenders for the establishment of a National Adolescent Health Network to facilitate the exchange of ideas, views and experience among a wide range of members; it is intended that this network will encourage objective evaluation of health promotion projects, disseminate information about effective health promotion and provide a means for young people themselves to comment on these activities.

In October, the Department for Education and Employment (DfEE) published a Health of the Nation/Health of the Young Nation wall-chart for schools, two free copies of which have been made available to schools on request. The DfEE and DH jointly published a handbook on child and adolescent mental health in April (see page 113)[7].

References

1. Department of Health. *The Health of the Nation: a strategy for health in England.* London: HMSO, 1992 (Cm. 1986).
2. Department of Health. *Fit for the future: second progress report on the Health of the Nation.* London: Department of Health, 1995.
3. Department of Health. *Policy appraisal and health: a guide from the Department of Health.* London: Department of Health, 1995.
4. Department of Health. *On the State of the Public Health: the report of the Chief Medical Officer of the Department of Health for the year 1993.* London: HMSO, 1994; 5, 74-112.
5. Department of Health. *Improving the health of mothers and children: NHS priorities for research and development: report to the NHS Central Research and Development Committee.* Leeds: Department of Health, 1995.
6. Department of Health. *Health of the Young Nation: your contribution counts.* London: Department of Health, 1995.
7. Department of Health, Social Services Inspectorate, Department for Education and Employment. *A handbook on child and adolescent mental health.* London: Department of Health, 1995.

(b)   Key areas and targets

(i)   *Coronary heart disease and stroke*

Over the years since the setting of the health strategy baseline[1], death rates for coronary heart disease (CHD) have fallen by an estimated 19.2% among people aged under 65 years and by about 12.5% among those aged 65-74 years; during the same period, stroke mortality fell by an estimated 8.5% for those aged under 65 years and by 14.3% for those aged 65-74 years.

Action to achieve the CHD/stroke targets[1] focused on physical activity, nutrition and obesity (see page 70), and smoking (see page 83). To assist those responsible for purchasing service interventions in these areas, the NHS Executive published *Assessing the options: CHD/stroke*[2] - an analysis of the target-effectiveness and cost-effectiveness of interventions to reduce CHD and stroke mortality.

The report of the 1993 Health Survey for England[3] was published in March and, for the third consecutive year, focused on CHD and its associated risk factors. New to the 1993 Survey was an analysis of the Dundee Risk Disk, which is suitable for use in general practice. This was used to assess the risk to individuals of overt CHD within the next 5 years: 14% of men and 15% of women aged 35-65 years were assessed to be at high risk, and 40% of men and 43% of women at intermediate risk. The health promotion scheme in general practice continued to emphasise broad population coverage; 94% of practices had achieved the highest level of health promotion actitivy (band 3) on 1 April 1995.

Inequalities in the use of health services between the sexes, indicated by the findings of the 1991 Health Survey[4], appear to persist with the 1993 finding[3] that 25% of men compared with 15% of women with a current cardiovascular condition had attended hospital in the previous 12 months as an outpatient for such a condition, and that 10% and 6%, respectively, had attended as an inpatient. Also, men were more likely (26%) than women (19%) to have had their serum cholesterol concentration measured at some time during their lives.

Work towards the development of a national strategy for physical activity continued with the Physical Activity Task Force's publication in May of *More people, more active, more often*[5]. This consultation document contained two major departures from previously accepted messages: firstly, that moderately intense physical activity is beneficial for cardiac health and, secondly, that the greatest public health gains will come from encouraging sedentary people to become more active at moderate intensity exercise. Based on these findings, DH commissioned the HEA to produce a national campaign to promote moderate physical activity for launch in Spring 1996. This campaign will include a focus on obesity, the development of which appears to be as much due to the lack of physical activity as to dietary factors.

Stroke was one of the first five topics chosen by the Central Health Outcomes Unit for the development of outcome measures. The Stroke Health Outcomes Group met for the first time in December, with wide representation from health professionals, health service management and the voluntary sector. The aim is to produce indicators to help to develop policy on health interventions and for the planning, developing and monitoring of services.

(ii)   Cancers

Breast cancer

The key intervention to reduce mortality from breast cancer is early detection through screening, to enable the provision of effective treatment at an earlier stage. In 1994/95, 976,300 women aged 50-64 years were screened; overall, 77.4% of women invited for screening took up their invitation. Of the 83 screening centres in England, 74 reported uptake of 70% (the target rate) or more. Four thousand nine hundred new cancers were detected, a rate of 5.0 per 1,000 women screened. Although this is a lower rate than in 1993/94, it reflects the fact that a substantially higher proportion of women screened were attending for a second or subsequent time; a lower cancer detection rate for these women (4.3 per 1,000) over those attending for the first time (5.5 per 1,000) was expected.

Cervical cancer

As for breast cancer, screening is the main intervention for cutting the incidence of cervical cancer by detection of early changes to the cervix that may lead to cancer, so enabling preventive treatment. In 1994/95, 3.9 million women were screened. At 31 March 1995, 85.7% of women aged 25-64 years resident in England had been screened at least once within the previous five years. Increasing uptake over recent years has been a very real achievement of the NHS cervical screening programme. The priority now is to achieve further improvements in screening quality; guidelines on new standards in quality assurance are expected to be published in Spring 1996.

Skin cancer

DH continued to fund the HEA's successful 'Sun Know How' campaign, which is aimed to make the public, especially people aged 8-30 years, more aware of actions that they should take to protect themselves against excessive exposure to ultraviolet (UV) radiation. The HEA and DH also work jointly to provide advice to colleges of further education that run fashion courses about features of clothing which reduce exposure to UV. The Department continued to fund the Meteorological Office to provide information for weather forecast presenters to broadcast as sunburn forecasts. Also, as part of the HEA campaign, information and warnings about sunburn were shown on the scoreboard during some cricket Test matches.

The Chief Medical Officer's 'Sun Challenge'[6], issued in February, sought assistance and support from the private sector and local authorities to get messages about safety in the sun over to the public. Towards the end of the year, the National Radiological Protection Board published a statement on the effects of UV radiation on human health[7]; guidelines on sunbed use were published by the Health and Safety Executive in October[8].

Knowledge, attitudes and behaviour in the sun have been monitored by the Office of Population Censuses and Surveys (OPCS, to become part of the Office for National Statistics [ONS] in Spring 1996): in the 12 months preceding October 1993, 37% of respondents to an OPCS survey had regretted at least one episode of sunburn, with the highest rates being found among people aged 16-24 years[9]; one-third of the respondents admitted that they had tried to get a tan. Two years later (in the 12 months preceding October 1995), the proportion who tried to get a tan was 39% - which indicates that a suntan is still considered to be desirable and that further work is needed in this area.

Lung cancer

Smoking remains by far the major risk-factor for lung cancer. Lung cancer is the most common cancer among males and the third most common in females (excluding non-melenoma skin cancers). The incidence of male lung cancer rises steeply with age from the mid-30s; it exceeds 560 per 100,000 population in men aged 70-74 years and exceeds 760 per 100,000 population in those aged 80-84 years. Overall, the current incidence among women is about 45% of that in men[10].

Awareness of the importance of smoking as the major risk-factor for lung cancer among the general population is now at a very high level. A recent survey by the HEA on knowledge, attitudes and behaviour[11] found that 96% of adults aged between 16 and 74 years quoted "giving up or cutting down on smoking" as a way to reduce the risk of getting lung cancer.

Adult cigarette smoking rates continue to fall: in 1994, some 28% of men smoked cigarettes compared with 29% in 1992; among women, 25% smoked in 1994 compared with 27% in 1992. Table 3.1 and Figure 3.1 show trends in adult smoking prevalence and the projected reduction required to meet the year 2000 target. Although it cannot be assumed that current trends will necessarily continue, the progress among adults is encouraging after the disappointing rise in cigarette smoking among secondary schoolchildren reported last year[12]. Cigarette consumption in the United Kingdom (UK) dropped from 98,000 million cigarettes in the year to June 1990 to 83,000 million cigarettes in the year to June 1995, against a target of 59,000 million by the year 2000.

In late 1994, the Government launched a three-year national anti-smoking campaign. During 1995, a new television advertising campaign was launched, supported by a new freephone number for the smoking Quitline and a range of local and national activities.

During 1995, the Scientific Committee on Tobacco and Health considered a number of areas including reviewing work on the health effects of exposure to environmental tobacco smoke.

(iii)   Mental illness

Progress continued to be made during 1995 to develop strategies to achieve the targets set under the mental illness key area of the strategy for health[1]. The focus

Table 3.1: *Prevalence of cigarette smoking among males and females aged 16 years and over, England, 1974-94*

Year	Males %	Females %	Total %
1974	51	40	45
1976	45	37	41
1978	44	36	40
1980	42	36	39
1982	37	32	35
1984	35	32	33
1986	34	31	32
1988	32	30	31
1990	31	28	29
1992	29	27	28
1994	28	25	26
2000 target	*20*	*20*	*20*

Note: Percentages rounded to nearest whole figure.

Source:OPCS/ONS (GHS)

Figure 3.1: *Prevalence of cigarette smoking among males and females aged 16 years and over, England, 1974-94, with health strategy target in 2000*

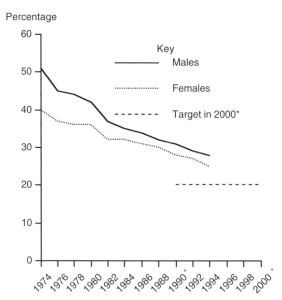

Note: *Baseline for Health of the Nation target of no more than 20% of adults smoking cigarettes in year 2000.

Source: OPCS/ONS (GHS)

of this work has been on the development and use of measures of the targets; related information collection; improved guidance to agencies and professionals within and outside the NHS, particularly with a view to improve purchasing of mental health services; and, for the longer term, the commissioning of further research.

The need for more detailed, systematic national data collection was identified after publication of the strategy. Data on the health and social functioning target were not readily available and the OPCS was commissioned to carry out the first national survey of psychiatric morbidity. The first three of eight full reports were published during the year[13,14,15]. These cover a survey of over 10,000 householders aged 16 to 64 years throughout Great Britain. Some of the findings are set out in the special chapter in this year's Report (see page 96). Other parts of the survey in preparation at the end of 1995 include a study of people receiving sheltered residential care and people who are homeless or have housing problems. Although the main focus is on health, social functioning, care received and mental health risk-factors, all respondents were also asked about suicidal ideas.

DH also commissioned research to compare the survey interview measure of psychiatric morbidity used in Great Britain with a similar structured interview used in other international studies, and during the year the development of the Health of the Nation outcome scale (HoNOS) was completed. This simple scale will help to measure improvements in the health and social functioning of mentally ill people; trials of its use in routine clinical practice and collection of these data through a new mental health minimum data set were carried out.

A number of systematic inquiries were completed during 1995. A study by the Clinical Standards Advisory Group on schizophrenia and severe mental illness[16], and a related study by the Social Services Inspectorate on implementation of the care programme approach for people in contact with specialist mental health services[17] revealed problems with the development of local, well-integrated specialised health and social care. In response to these findings, the Secretary of State for Health set up an inquiry by the NHS Executive into the purchasing of mental health services in England by local health authorities, and a booklet on the spectrum of care and available services was prepared for distribution to patients in every district. The Mental Health (Patients in the Community) Act 1995[18] received Royal Assent on 8 November. It introduces, from 1 April 1996, 'supervised discharge' for a limited number of patients who have been detained for treatment under the Mental Health Act 1983[19] and are ready to leave hospital, but who would present a particular risk to themselves or other people if they did not receive proper care. These patients can now be placed under formal supervision to help to ensure that they receive the services they need in the community.

During 1995, mental health was listed as one of the NHS's six medium-term priorities in its 1996/97 *Priorities and planning guidance*[20], emphasising the importance of mental health to health authorities and NHS Trusts. Routine monitoring of the implementation of the care programme approach showed that all districts had established a supervision register to identify to staff those patients at the greatest risk of self-neglect or harm to self or others, to ensure more effective support and supervision of such patients after discharge from inpatient care. *Building bridges*[21], with useful guidance on inter-Agency collaboration and on implementation of the care programme approach, was published in October. A series of regional workshops on housing and mental illness was conducted jointly with the Department of the Environment (DoE), and close collaboration between health care and social services support for community care for people with severe mental health problems was provided through the continuation of the mental illness specific grant and the mentally ill initiative.

Mental health was the first major topic in the national NHS research and development programme, and the first reports on methods for individual and population-based mental health needs assessment became available in March[22]. As part of the Department's concordat with the Medical Research Council, a review was published on the scope for research on suicide reduction[23]; it was agreed that, after 18 months, the success of this initiative in triggering new research projects would be reviewed.

A sub-group of the Wider Health Working Group was established to advise on how to reduce suicide rates among the general population through measures to reduce access to readily available means of suicide, by changing public attitudes and by the development of specific strategies for high-risk groups. Over the four years since the health strategy baseline was set, suicide death rates dropped by nearly 8%.

(iv) HIV/AIDS and sexual health

The Health of the Nation[1] objectives for HIV/AIDS and sexual health are to reduce the incidence of HIV infection and other sexually transmitted diseases (STDs) and to reduce unwanted pregnancies. In 1995/96, DH allocated £244.7 million to health authorities in England towards HIV treatment costs, including £49 million to prevent the spread of HIV infection by public education, protection of the blood supply, provision of testing facilities and staff training. Also in 1995/96, £13.4 million were allocated to local authorities, £1.5 million to voluntary organisations and £5.8 million to the HEA and the National AIDS/Drugs Helpline.

In 1993, conceptions among girls aged under 16 years fell by 5%, following falls of 10% in 1992 and 7% in 1991; this decrease appears to be reversing the rising trend throughout the 1980s.

In March, the Department launched the 'Sexwise' campaign which offers young people a free, confidential phoneline and the opportunity to talk to a trained adviser about sex and personal relationships. Radio advertisements concentrated on the London and Manchester areas, and led to over 330,000 calls in the first year of operation. A second round of publicity is planned for Trent and the North-East for Spring 1996.

(v)   Accidents

Encouraging progress continues to be made towards the Health of the Nation targets[1] for reductions in accident mortality. Over the four years since the health strategy baselines were set, death rates from accidents have fallen by over 30% among children aged under 15 years, and by about 25% in those aged 15-24 years. Among those aged over 65 years, a smaller fall of some 6% has been seen, although changes in the assignment of deaths from osteoporosis may have led to underestimation of this fall.

The Accident Prevention Task Force - which includes representatives from eight Government Departments, local authorities, the police, voluntary organisations, schools and universities, nursing and industry - continued to address information and research needs.

A review[24] of the causes and relative risks of accidents relevant to the Health of the Nation targets, commissioned by DH and published in June, was distributed to environmental health officers, road safety officers and others involved in accident prevention. It assessed the research evidence of the efficacy, effectiveness, cost-effectiveness and appropriateness of different interventions to prevent or minimise injury from accidents, and the available outcome and process measures to monitor the Health of the Nation accident targets.

A report by the DH Public Health Information Strategy (PHIS) team[25] described and assessed accident data collection by various bodies such as the police, the Department of Trade and Industry and the fire services in place in 1993, and identified the need for a more comprehensive framework for collecting information on accidents; this report was distributed by DH in January. A second report of the PHIS team[26] to describe the opportunities for linking and sharing data between existing sources and to set standards for future development was accepted by the Task Force at a meeting in December, and will be distributed in Summer, 1996. In addition, the 1995 Health Survey for England included coverage of accidental injuries in the population-based study.

An overview of effective interventions to prevent accidents among adolescents[27] will be distributed to statutory and voluntary organisations early in 1996. In May, DH distributed the Medical Commission on Accident Prevention's updated book *Medical aspects of fitness to drive: a guide for medical practitioners*[28]. Changes in the regulations on epilepsy and driving, and a section on drugs and driving, were included.

Public awareness about child accident prevention was raised through the 'Child Safety Week' campaign, an annual event co-ordinated by the Child Accident Prevention Trust. The campaign showed inter-Departmental co-ordination, with support and funding from the Departments of Transport and Trade and Industry and the Department for Education and Employment (DfEE).

References

1. Department of Health. *The Health of the Nation: a strategy for health in England.* London: HMSO, 1992 (Cm. 1986).
2. Department of Health. *Assessing the options: CHD/stroke: target-effectiveness and cost-effectiveness of interventions to reduce CHD and stroke mortality.* London: Department of Health, 1995.
3. Bennett N, Dodd T, Flatley J, Freeth S, Bolling K. *Health Survey for England 1993.* London: HMSO, 1995 (Series HS; no. 3).
4. White A, Nicolaas G, Foster K, Browne F, Carey S. *Health Survey for England 1991: a survey carried out by the Social Survey Division of OPCS on behalf of the Department of Health.* London: HMSO, 1993 (Series HS; no. 1).
5. Physical Activity Task Force, Department of Health. *More people, more active, more often: physical activity in England: a consultation paper.* London: Department of Health, 1995.
6. Department of Health. *Sun challenge.* Wetherby (West Yorkshire): Department of Health, 1995.
7. National Radiological Protection Board. *Board statement on effects of ultraviolet radiation on human health and health effects from ultraviolet radiation: report of an Advisory Group on Non-Ionising Radiation.* Didcot (Oxon): National Radiological Protection Board, 1995 (*Doc NRPB* vol. 6 no. 2).
8. Health and Safety Executive. *Controlling health risks from the use of UV tanning equipment.* London: Health and Safety Executive, 1995.
9. Melia J, Bulman A. Sunburn and tanning in a British population. *J Public Health Med* 1995; **17**: 223-9.
10. Office of Population Censuses and Surveys. *Registrations of cancer diagnosed in 1990, England and Wales.* London: Office of Population Censuses and Surveys, 1995 (Series MB1 95/1).
11. Office for National Statistics, Social Survey Division. *Health in England 1995: what people know, what people think, what people do: a survey of adults aged 16-74 in England carried out by the Social Survey Division of ONS on behalf of the Health Education Authority.* London: HMSO (in press).
12. Department of Health. *On the State of the Public Health: the annual report of the Chief Medical Officer of the Department of Health for the year 1994.* London: HMSO, 1994; 65-8, 79.
13. Meltzer H, Gill B, Petticrew M, Hinds K. *The prevalence of psychiatric morbidity among adults living in private households.* London: Office of Population Censuses and Surveys, 1995 (OPCS Surveys of Psychiatric Morbidity in Great Britain; bulletin no. 2).
14. Meltzer H, Gill B, Petticrew M, Hinds K. *Physical complaints, service use and treatment of adults with psychiatric disorders.* London: HMSO, 1995 (OPCS Surveys of Psychiatric Morbidity in Great Britain; report no. 2).
15. Meltzer H, Gill B, Petticrew M, Hinds K. *Economic activity and social functioning of adults with psychiatric disorders.* London: HMSO 1995 (OPCS Surveys of Psychiatric Morbidity in Great Britain; report no. 3).
16. Clinical Standards Advisory Group, Department of Health. *Schizophrenia: vols 1 and 2: report of a CSAG committee on schizophrenia.* London: HMSO, 1995.
17. Department of Health. *Social services departments and the care programme approach: an inspection.* London: Department of Health, 1995.
18. *The Mental Health (Patients in the Community) Act 1995.* London: HMSO, 1995.
19. *The Mental Health Act 1983.* London: HMSO, 1983.
20. NHS Executive. *Priorities and planning guidance for the NHS: 1996/97.* Wetherby (West Yorkshire): Department of Health, 1995.
21. Department of Health. *Building bridges: a guide to arrangements for inter-Agency working for the care and protection of severely mentally ill people.* London: Department of Health, 1995. (OPCS Surveys of Psychiatric Morbidity in Great Britain; bulletin no. 2).
22. Stevens A, Raftery J, eds. *Health care needs assessment: the epidemiologically based needs assessment reviews: mental illness.* Oxford: Radcliffe Medical Press, 1994.
23. Confidential Inquiry into Homicides and Suicides by Mentally Ill People. *Report of the Confidential Inquiry into Homicides and Suicides by Mentally Ill People.* London: Royal College of Psychiatrists (in press).
24. Higginson I. *Health of the Nation accident reduction targets: a research review: what further work is needed?* London: Department of Health, 1995.
25. Department of Health. *Improving information on accidents.* London: Department of Health, 1993 (Public Health Information Strategy; Implementation Project no. 19).

26. Department of Health. *Agreeing an accident information strategy*. London: Department of Health, 1995 (Public Health Information Strategy; Implementation Project no. 19B).
27. Coleman P, Munro J, Nicholl J, Harper R, Kent G, Wild D. *The effectiveness of interventions to prevent accidental injury to adolescents and young people aged 15-24 years: a review of the evidence*. Sheffield: Medical Care Research Unit, University of Sheffield (in press).
28. Taylor JF, ed. *Medical aspects of fitness to drive: a guide for medical practitioners, 5th edn.* London: Medical Commission on Accident Prevention, 1995.

(c)   Variations in health

The 1994 Report[1] drew attention to the way in which variations in health are associated with gender, social class, geography, ethnicity and occupation. Such variations have been observed for more than a century. However, whilst socio-economic, gender, regional and ethnic differences are widespread and are observable in all countries, the magnitude of these differences is not fixed; differences are recorded within and between countries and over different time periods, indicating that some variations at least are susceptible to change through intervention.

In 1994, the Chief Medical Officer set up a Working Group to report on how DH and the NHS could tackle variations in health in the Health of the Nation key areas[2], and on what further research was needed. The Group's report[3] was published in October 1995, and was widely distributed to health and local authorities and others (see page 66). The Working Group found that a considerable amount of activity was taking place within the NHS to try to tackle variations in health, but that much of this work was at the margins of health authority activity and little of it was being evaluated. A study was commissioned from the Centre for Reviews and Dissemination at York University to review what health interventions had been demonstrated to be effective.

This study[4] showed that the available evidence on effectiveness was very limited and that there is a pressing need for more, and more rigorous, evaluation of interventions. The report's main recommendations were that:

—   health authorities and general practitioner (GP) purchasers should have a plan to identify and tackle variations and to evaluate interventions;

—   such a plan should include provision for working in alliance with other relevant bodies;

—   health authorities, GP purchasers and NHS Trusts should take steps to monitor access to services, to safeguard equitable access;

—   DH should work actively in alliance with other Government Departments and other bodies to encourage social policies which promote health; hold the NHS to account for implementation of the recommendations applying to the NHS; and take forward the report's recommendations on research;

—   health authority purchasers should undertake rigorous evaluations of interventions which they implement;

— health authority purchasers should be supported in the task of evaluation by the establishment of a clearing house;

— the MRC, Economic and Social Research Council and DH should co-ordinate their programmes of research; *and*

— a DH research consultation exercise should recommend priorities for the evaluation of interventions to address health variations, research to address the needs of particularly vulnerable groups of the population, and basic research into causal processes.

A £2.4 million research initiative will be launched in 1996, drawing on the outcome of the consultation exercise recommended by the Working Group, which was completed at the end of 1995.

References

1. Department of Health. *On the State of the Public Health: the annual report of the Chief Medical Officer of the Department of Health for the year 1994.* London: HMSO, 1995; 64-5.
2. Department of Health. *The Health of the Nation: a strategy for health in England.* London: Department of Health, 1992 (Cm. 1986).
3. Department of Health. *Variations in health: what can the Department of Health and the NHS do?* London: Department of Health, 1995.
4. NHS Centre for Reviews and Dissemination, University of York. *Review of research on the effectiveness of health service interventions to reduce variations in health.* York: NHS Centre for Reviews and Dissemination, University of York, 1995 (CRD report, no.3).

(d)   Implementation

(i)   *Priorities for the NHS*

The strategic goal of improving health through the Health of the Nation initiative[1] was identified as a top objective for the NHS in its *Priorities and planning guidance* for 1994/95[2] and 1995/96[3], and continues to provide the main context for NHS planning[4]. Since its launch in 1992, the strategy has had an increasing influence on health authorities' plans to purchase services to meet the health care needs of local people. It has also encouraged the formation of health alliances with a variety of local organisations to improve health. Most Directors of Public Health (DsPH) now feature the initiative prominently in their annual reports on the health of local populations, and corporate contracts ensure that health authorities, hospital and community services and primary care teams deliver suitable local programmes supported by management action.

The NHS Executive met representatives of all the health regions in the Summer of 1994 to discuss and agree regional targets; aggregation of these indicated that the NHS was confident of achieving the vast majority of these targets, and good progress has since been made in most areas.

The NHS Executive is developing a performance management framework for the Health of the Nation initiative with Regional Offices and health authorities. This framework uses a variety of performance management indicators developed to take local circumstances into account. Increasingly, public health and performance management teams are working closely together to review progress towards Health of the Nation targets as part of the normal performance management process. Some performance indicators feature in quarterly progress reports to the NHS Executive Board. A small number of carefully chosen indicators will be added to the Common Information Core in April 1996, which will monitor progress across key areas. This work will supplement extensive existing NHS public health action, such as local monitoring of the speed with which patients receive thrombolytic treatment after myocardial infarction.

The NHS Executive, working closely with local colleagues, has a project team to provide practical help and support for the NHS on implementation of the Health of the Nation strategy. A project steering board, which reports to the Chief Executive's Health of the Nation Working Group (both of which have NHS representation), co-ordinates and supports such implementation under three main project headings (purchasing, providing and primary care), with supporting work on communications, management information, research and development, and education and training. These groups both have an important role in co-ordination with the wider Department and ensuring that the NHS has an early input into the development of policy. A practical example is the health promoting hospitals initiative, which has provided a framework for a wide range of health promotion initiatives.

(ii)   Local health alliances

The Health of the Nation White Paper[1] identified health alliances as a powerful tool for delivering health gain and working towards its targets. Indeed, nationally the strategy is led by a Cabinet sub-committee, chaired by the Lord President of the Council, which steers the strategy as an alliance between Government Departments.

To encourage the formation of local health alliances, the Health Alliance Awards Scheme was developed. This competition runs at regional and at national levels, which culminated this year in an awards ceremony in London in April, with prizes for the best alliances working in each of the five key areas, for an alliance whose work spanned two or more of the key areas, and for an alliance of national organisations.

This awards scheme was a great success. Attention was drawn to a great diversity of alliances working in many very different areas; a lot of them were targeted at groups of people who can easily be overlooked or slip through more conventional communications and health care systems. The best of the alliances developed sophisticated and effective means to evaluate their work, and the awards scheme allowed their efforts to be recognised publicly and held up as good practice for others to follow. A guide to the evaluation of alliances was also published[5]. The second year of the awards scheme has introduced a new category for alliances whose work focuses on young people to support the Health of the Young Nation initiative. By the closing date of 31 October, 300 entries had been received, indicating a continued high level of interest.

(iii) **Healthy settings**

By the introduction of the concept of healthy settings, the Health of the Nation initiative[1] emphasised that responsibility for health, and influences on health, extend far beyond DH and the NHS. The healthy settings (cities, schools, hospitals, the workplace, homes, prisons and the environment) cast their collective net so wide that they cover the entire population, often several times over.

Health in the workplace featured as the special chapter in last year's Report[6], and is reviewed again on page 75. Good progress was made in the European network of health promoting schools. Within this project there are 16 pilot schools (seven secondary, six primary and three special), each matched against two reference schools; each pilot school receives support towards becoming a health promoting school, and evaluation of progress in the pilot and reference schools will be completed in 1997. A report of a baseline survey of health promotion attitudes and activities in more than 500 schools was published in October by the HEA[7]. DH links with the UK Health for All Network, the co-ordinating body for healthy cities projects, were reinforced and developed; the Department was represented at the Network's annual general meeting in November. 'City Challenge' and the single regeneration budget, both administered by the DoE, are contributing to health promotion initiatives and the development of local partnerships. Dr John Chalstrey, the Lord Mayor of London for 1995-96, has chosen 'Good Health to the City and the Nation' as the theme for his year of office. This links with several of the healthy settings, including the workplace, and DH has supplied a secondee to help the Lord Mayor to develop this theme. The Prison Service Directorate of the Home Office is working with the World Health Organization on the possibility of becoming a collaborating centre for healthy prisons (see page 154).

(iv) **Inter-Departmental co-operation**

A great deal of the work in the healthy settings relies on the co-operation of other Government Departments. Healthy environment, for instance, falls to the DoE. Its policies to maintain and improve the quality of drinking water and to improve the quality of bathing water are clearly important to maintain and to improve health. In January, the DoE published its strategic policies for air quality management in *Air quality: meeting the challenge*[8]; amendments have been introduced to the Environment Bill to provide a statutory framework for implementation of these policies.

In October, the DfEE launched a free wall-chart with key facts for schools about the Health of the Nation initiative, which was sent to chief education officers and advertised in the DfEE's *Schools' Update*. DH also sent copies to regional and district DsPH (see page 71).

The Ministry of Agriculture, Fisheries and Food (MAFF) is involved in four of the five key areas, but primarily with CHD and stroke. It is jointly responsible, with DH, for overseeing the implementation and monitoring of the Nutrition Task Force programme of action *Eat well!*[9], with particular responsibility for aspects that involve the food chain. The MAFF provides support to the programme in research on the links between diet and health and the influences on consumer choice; national surveillance of the diet and the nutritional health of the population (via the MAFF National Food Survey); information on the nutritional content of food; and information and advice to consumers. The MAFF is helping to promote awareness of the problem of mental health issues among farmers and of the services available to assist those in distress, and to raise awareness of the need for care to reduce the level of accidents on farms.

DH also maintains close links with the HSE to co-ordinate health promotion efforts in the workplace. The HSE's campaign 'Good health is good business' complements the Department's own workplace health promotion initiative.

The Department of Transport continues to contribute to the accidents key area through its work to reduce road traffic accidents; its work to promote cycling and walking also relates to the physical activity aspect of the CHD and stroke prevention key area.

References

1. Department of Health. *The Health of the Nation: a strategy for health in England.* London: HMSO, 1992 (Cm. 1986).
2. NHS Executive. *Priorities and planning guidance for the NHS 1994/95.* Leeds: Department of Health, 1993 (Executive Letter: EL(93)54).
3. NHS Executive. *Priorities and planning guidance for the NHS 1995/96.* Leeds: Department of Health, 1994 (Executive Letter: EL(94)55).
4. NHS Executive. *Priorities and planning guidance for the NHS 1996/97.* Wetherby (West Yorkshire): Department of Health, 1995 (Executive Letter: EL(95)68).
5. Funnel R, Oldfield K, Speller V. *Towards healthier alliances: a tool for planning, evaluating and developing healthier alliances.* London: Health Education Authority, 1995.
6. Department of Health. *On the State of the Public Health: the annual report of the Chief Medical Officer of the Department of Health for the year 1994.* London: HMSO, 1995: 7, 88-127.
7. Health Education Authority, National Foundation for Educational Research in England and Wales. *The health promoting school: a baseline survey.* London: Health Education Authority, 1995.
8. Department of the Environment, Air Quality Division. *Air quality: meeting the challenge: the Government's strategic policies for air-quality management.* London: Department of the Environment, 1995.
9. Department of Health, Nutrition Task Force. *Eat well! An action plan from the Nutrition Task Force to achieve the Health of the Nation targets on diet and nutrition.* London: Department of Health, 1994.

(e)   The way ahead

The Health of the Nation communications team continues to play a key role in keeping all participants informed about progress, developments and events in the strategy for health. *Target*, the Health of the Nation newsletter, continues to be published regularly, with contributions from its wide readership. The Health of the Nation calendar, launched in 1995, has been well received and, in response to requests, a briefing pack will be produced early in 1996.

Much current work is cumulative and long-term; most targets fall due in the year 2000 or beyond, and some health promotion activities (eg, on nutrition and physical activity) with young people will not show their true value for many years to come. For these reasons, it is particularly important to develop the best possible tools to monitor the effects of interventions.

As indicated by the Health of the Nation White Paper[1], the health of an individual is dependent at least in part on their own lifestyle and behaviour. An understanding of health-related behaviours and the factors which influence them is essential to the success of the health strategy. DH has therefore set up research into behavioural epidemiology, which will include reviews of existing knowledge - for example, an epidemiological overview on how health-related behaviours relevant to the five key areas are distributed across time, place and person. This overview will be published early in 1996 at around the same time as the fourth report of the Health Survey for England and the report of the HEA's Health Education Monitoring Survey. The three reports will be complementary, and together will help to identify particular sub-groups in the population who may be at increased risk, to recognise specific gaps in knowledge and to generate hypotheses which may then be tested through further research.

Reference

1. Department of Health: *The Health of the Nation: a strategy for health in England.* London: HMSO, 1992 (Cm. 1986).

CHAPTER 4

MENTAL HEALTH

(a)   Introduction

The Department of Health (DH) has set an evidence-based mental health strategy for England, which encompasses where and how people are cared for, and with what aims and goals in view. This strategy should ensure that policy is well rooted in the known epidemiology of mental disorders; that policy does not only focus on those patients with severe mental disorders who need specialist care, but also on those with less severe disorders in primary care, in schools, in the workplace and in prisons; that there is effective integration of mental health services with other agencies; that mental health care policies are rooted in a coherent framework of prevention and mental health promotion; and that the effects of such policies are measured by health and social outcomes as well as by statistics which reflect the use of mental health services.

DH's objectives for mental illness are:

— to reduce the incidence and prevalence of mental disorder;

— to reduce the mortality (both from suicide and from deaths from physical illness) associated with mental disorder;

— to reduce the extent and severity of other problems associated with mental disorders, such as poor physical health, impaired psychological and social functioning, poor social circumstances and family burden;

— to ensure delivery of appropriate services and interventions;

— to reverse the public's negative perceptions of mental illness by countering fear, ignorance and stigma, creating a more positive social climate in which people are encouraged rather than deterred from seeking help, and improving the quality of life for people with mental health problems; *and*

— to research the causes, consequences and care of specific mental disorders.

In 1992, the Government published *The Health of the Nation* White Paper[1], which set out a strategic framework for the achievement of health gain in five key areas, one of which was mental illness[2], and set targets for the prevention of morbidity and mortality. The targets for mental illness are shown on page 125. The framework to achieve these targets involves the improvement of information and understanding, the development of comprehensive local services and the general encouragement of good practice.

References

1. Department of Health. *The Health of the Nation: a strategy for health in England.* London: HMSO, 1992 (Cm. 1986).
2. Department of Health. *The mental illness key area handbook, 2nd edn.* London: HMSO, 1994.

(b)   Information about mental illness

Monitoring the state of public mental health, planning the nature and volumes of services likely to be required and evaluating the effectiveness of services provided all depend on reliable information. In the light of the Health of the Nation targets[1], and the broader aims they reflect, the scope and nature of information collection is being comprehensively reviewed and upgraded.

(i)   Epidemiology of mental disorders

Adults

An extensive two-phase epidemiological survey of psychiatric morbidity throughout Great Britain has been carried out by the Office of Population Censuses and Surveys (OPCS, which will become part of the Office for National Statistics [ONS] from Spring 1996) and an advisory group of psychiatric epidemiologists in samples from households, institutions and among homeless people[2,3,4,5,6,7,8,9]. The survey was commissioned by DH, the Welsh Office and the Scottish Home and Health Department to give a national picture of the prevalence, severity and duration of mental disorders and their accompanying social disability (and thereby to give a baseline measure of the first Health of the Nation mental health target); associated risk-factors; and the extent to which health and social care needs are met by services. This is the first national survey in any country to collect data on prevalence, risk-factors, and associated disability simultaneously in household, institutional and homeless samples by use of standardised assessment techniques. Most of the disorders in the Health of the Nation target are covered - principally neuroses, affective disorders and psychoses. Similar surveys of children, adolescents, elderly people and of individuals held in custody are planned. The Department has also commissioned a psychiatric validation study within the fourth national survey of ethnic minorities.

The OPCS surveys revealed that one in six adults aged 16 to 64 years who are living in private households had suffered from some type of neurotic disorder in the week before the survey interview, half of which was mixed anxiety-depressive disorder. All types of neurotic disorders were more common among women than men. Marital status was strongly associated with neurotic disorder; rates were substantially higher in separated, divorced and widowed individuals of both genders and among co-habiting women. Unemployed people were about twice as likely to suffer neurotic disorders compared with people in work; those living in urban settings were 1.5 times as likely to suffer them than rural dwellers. Table 4.1 shows socio-demographic associations of a raised total Clinical Interview Schedule (CIS-R) score, based on multiple logistic regression analysis. Table 4.2 shows how the prevalence of neurotic disorders, psychosis, drug and alcohol dependence varies according to economic activity, with data compiled separately for men and women.

Table 4.1: *Odds ratios (ORs) of socio-demographic associations of Clinical Interview Schedule (CIS-R) score, Great Britain, 1993*

CIS-R score of 12 or more		Adjusted OR	95% CI
Sex	Male	1.00	-
	Female	1.56*	1.37, 1.78
Age (years)	16-24	1.00	-
	25-34	1.07	0.87, 1.32
	35-44	1.23	0.99, 1.53
	45-54	1.24	0.99, 1.55
	55-64	0.72*	0.56, 0.91
Family unit type	Couple: no children	1.00	-
	Couple: 1 + child	1.03	0.87, 1.21
	Lone parent + child	1.56*	1.26, 1.93
	One person only	1.48*	1.25, 1.76
	Adult with parents	0.76	0.54, 1.05
	Adult with one parent	0.80	0.54, 1.19
Employment status	Working full time	1.00	-
	Working part-time	1.19	1.00, 1.42
	Unemployed	2.26*	1.87, 2.72
	Economically inactive	1.71*	1.47, 2.00
Accommodation	Detached	1.00	-
	Semi-detached	0.96	0.80, 1.15
	Terraced	1.19	1.00, 1.43
	Flat/maisonette	1.15	0.93, 1.43
Tenure	Owner/occupier	1.00	-
	Renter	1.33*	1.16, 1.53
Locality	Semi-rural/rural	1.00	-
	Urban	1.21*	1.06, 1.38

CI = Confidence interval.
*p<0.01.

Source: OPCS/ONS

About half of individuals identified as having a neurotic disorder suffered from long-standing physical complaints compared with 30% of other individuals. This differential was seen across all ages and both genders. Individuals with neuroses were twice as likely as those without to have consulted their general practitioner (GP) in the fortnight before interview. However, one-quarter of those with a neurotic disorder had not consulted any professional about their mental health, usually because they thought no one could help. Figure 4.1 shows a profile of health service use in the previous year among people with neurotic disorders; Figure 4.2 shows prevalence (and prevalence by gender) of neurotic disorders.

Figure 4.1: *Profile of health service use in previous year among people with neurotic disorders, Great Britain, 1993*

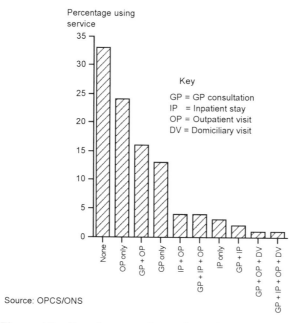

Source: OPCS/ONS

Figure 4.2: *Prevalence, and prevalence by sex, of neurotic disorders, adults aged 16-64 years living in private households, Great Britain, 1993*

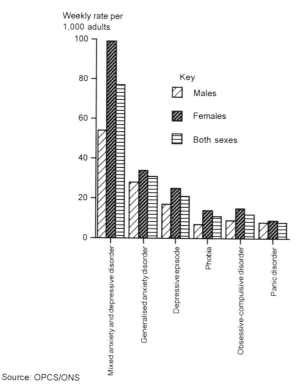

Source: OPCS/ONS

Table 4.2: *Prevalence of psychiatric disorders per 1,000 population by economic activity and sex, adults aged 16-64 years, Great Britain, 1993*

	Employment status								All	
	Working full-time		Working part-time		Unemployed		Economic inactive			

Women

Rate per 1,000 in past week *SE*

Mixed anxiety and depressive disorder	94	8	88	8	206	27	94	8	99	5
Generalised anxiety disorder	29	4	27	5	60	15	41	4	34	3
Depressive episode	11	2	22	4	56	13	37	5	25	2
All phobias	8	2	12	3	23	10	22	4	14	2
Obsessive-compulsive disorder	13	3	13	3	27	10	16	3	15	2
Panic disorder	9	3	7	3	9	4	10	2	9	1
Any neurotic disorder	164	11	168	11	381	34	220	11	195	7

Rate per 1,000 in past 12 months *SE*

Functional psychoses	2	1	4	2	10	5	7	2	5	1
Alcohol dependence	18	3	31	6	28	14	18	4	22	2
Drug dependence	7	2	11	3	55	14	20	4	15	2

Men

Rate per 1,000 in past week *SE*

Mixed anxiety and depressive disorder	46	4	56	16	80	12	76	11	54	4
Generalised anxiety disorder	21	3	29	17	51	10	37	7	28	2
Depressive episode	12	2	16	10	27	8	37	8	17	2
All phobias	4	1	5	4	17	6	14	4	7	1
Obsessive-compulsive disorder	7	1	6	5	16	5	20	6	9	2
Panic disorder	6	2	5	5	12	6	12	4	8	2
Any neurotic disorder	95	6	117	25	203	18	195	18	123	5

Rate per 1,000 in past 12 months *SE*

Functional psychoses	2	1	10	8	6	3	14	5	4	1
Alcohol dependence	74	6	91	21	117	16	56	10	77	5
Drug dependence	15	3	51	17	96	16	29	6	29	3

All adults

Rate per 1,000 in past week *SE*

Mixed anxiety and depressive disorder	62	4	83	7	120	13	89	7	77	3
Generalised anxiety disorder	24	3	27	5	54	9	40	4	31	2
Depressive episode	11	1	21	4	36	6	37	4	21	1
All phobias	5	1	11	3	19	5	20	3	11	1
Obsessive-compulsive disorder	9	1	12	3	19	5	17	3	12	1
Panic disorder	7	1	7	2	11	4	11	2	8	1
Any neurotic disorder	118	6	160	10	259	17	212	10	160	5

Rate per 1,000 in past 12 months *SE*

Functional psychoses	2	1	5	2	7	2	9	2	4	1
Alcohol dependence	54	4	42	6	89	13	29	4	49	3
Drug dependence	13	2	17	4	83	12	23	3	22	2

SE = Standard error of the mean.

Source: OPCS/ONS

Table 4.3: *Type of medication by number of neurotic disorders, adults aged 16-64 years, Great Britain, 1993*

	Number of disorders		
	One neurotic disorder	Two or more disorders	Any neurotic disorder
Percentage of adults taking each type of medication			
Any antidepressant	62	74	67
Tricyclic antidepressants	48	48	48
Monoamine oxidase inhibitors	1	1	1
Compound antidepressants	-	-	-
Other antidepressants	13	25	18
Any anxiolytic or hypnotic	47	49	48
Anxiolytics	22	35	27
Hypnotics	26	20	24
Base (= people on medication)	*81*	*52*	*133*

Source: OPCS/ONS

Table 4.4: *Type of therapy or counselling by number of neurotic disorders, adults aged 16-64 years, Great Britain, 1993*

	Number of disorders		
	One neurotic disorder	Two or more disorders	Any neurotic disorder
Percentage of adults with each type of treatment			
Psychotherapy, psychoanalysis, individual or group therapy etc	41	9	39
Behaviour or cognitive therapy	2	-	2
Sex, marital or family therapy	3	-	2
Art, music or drama therapy	2	-	2
Social skills training	3	3	5
Counselling	48	15	51
Base (=people having therapy or counselling)	*65*	*25*	*91*

Source: OPCS/ONS

Table 4.5: *Odds ratios (ORs) associated with treatment by antidepressants, adults aged 16-64 years, Great Britain, 1993*

Factors	Adjusted ORs	95% CI
Number of neurotic disorders		
One	1.00	-
Two or more	4.85	3.04, 7.73
Age (years)		
16-24	1.00	-
25-34	1.49	0.60, 3.71
35-44	2.66	1.12, 6.33
45-54	3.19	1.37, 7.47
55-64	1.86	0.73, 4.74
Employment status		
Working full-time	1.00	-
Working part-time	0.93	0.42, 2.07
Unemployed	1.27	0.58, 2.78
Economically inactive	2.35	1.32, 4.13
Physical illness		
No	1.00	-
Yes	1.62	1.00, 2.64

CI = Confidence interval.

Source: OPCS/ONS

Tables 4.3 and 4.4 show the relation between the number of neurotic disorders suffered and the type of medication and of therapy or counselling received. Table 4.3 shows that medication is more likely to be in the form of an antidepressant than an anxiolytic. Table 4.4 indicates that counselling is the commonest form of talking treatment received. Table 4.5 shows that antidepressants are more likely to be prescribed to adults with two or more disorders, to those aged 35-54 years, to the economically inactive and to those who are also physically ill. Table 4.6 shows the factors which influence who is treated with anxiolytics or hypnotics.

Subjects with significant depressive symptoms were asked about suicidal ideas. Just under 1% of the total sample in the OPCS survey reported suicidal thoughts in the preceding week, two-thirds of them women. One-fifth of those reporting suicidal ideas were receiving antidepressant medication and one-sixth were receiving counselling or psychotherapy. One adult in 20 had experienced symptoms of alcohol dependence in the preceding year and one in 40 dependence on drugs. Men were over three times as likely as women to be dependent on alcohol and twice as likely to be dependent on drugs (see Figure 4.3). Alcohol dependence was nearly twice as common among those who were unemployed compared with those who were working; drug dependence was over five times more frequent among unemployed people.

Table 4.6: *Odds ratios (ORs) associated with treatment by anxiolytics or hypnotics, adults aged 16-64 years, Great Britain, 1993*

Factors	Adjusted ORs	95% CI
Number of neurotic disorders		
One	1.00	-
Two or more	4.04	2.32, 7.04
Age (years)		
16-24	1.00	-
25-34	1.04	0.20, 5.44
35-44	4.78	1.10, 20.68
45-54	7.50	1.76, 32.00
55-64	8.93	2.04, 38.98
Family type		
Couple no child	1.00	-
Couple and child(ren)	0.70	0.32, 1.54
Lone parent and child(ren)	1.40	0.51, 3.82
One person only	2.79	1.40, 5.59
Adult with parents	2.32	0.39, 13.69
Adult with one parent	0.86	0.05, 15.74
Physical illness		
No	1.00	-
Yes	2.42	1.31, 4.51

CI = Confidence interval.

Source: OPCS/ONS

Figure 4.3: *Prevalence of alcohol and drug dependence by sex, adults aged 16-64 years, Great Britain, 1993*

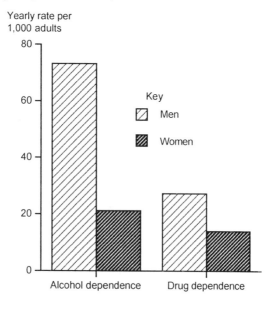

Source: OPCS/ONS

Table 4.7: *Economic activity of adults with a psychotic disorder, a neurotic disorder and no psychiatric disorder, Great Britain, 1993*

	Adults with a psychotic disorder	Adults with a neurotic disorder	All with no psychiatric disorder
	%	%	%
Working	39	56	71
Looking for work	11	11	7
Intending to look, temporarily sick	2	2	2
Permanently unable to work	21	12	2
Retired	10	2	4
Full time education	5	4	4
Keeping house	9	13	10
Other	2	1	1
Base	*44*	*1557*	*8184*

Source: OPCS/ONS

Table 4.8: *Financial position of adults with a psychotic disorder, a neurotic disorder and no psychiatric disorder, Great Britain, 1993*

	Adults with a psychotic disorder	Adults with a neurotic disorder	All adults surveyed in 1993 for the GHS/Omnibus Surveys[*]
State benefits	*Percentage receiving each State benefit*		
Income support	31	19	10
Invalidity pension, benefit or allowance	17	9	2
Sickness benefit	11	3	0
Disability living allowance	7	2	2
Attendance allowance	5	1	-
Base	*44*	*1557*	*13744*
Personal income	*Mid-point of income band*		
Median, weekly gross income	£90	£90	£150
Base	*44*	*1557*	*18760*

[*] State benefits data from GHS; Income data from Omnibus Survey.

Source: OPCS/ONS

Functional psychoses carry an even higher risk than neuroses of a chronic disabling course, and thus incidence and prevalence differ considerably. The OPCS national survey indicated that the overall prevalence of psychosis (mainly schizophrenia and affective disorders) was four per 1,000, with that for urban dwellers being twice that for those living in the country. Of people with psychosis, two-thirds were in touch with specialist services, whilst 18% had seen only their GP in the year before interview and a further 18% claimed never to have sought professional help.

Table 4.9: *Participation in outdoor and indoor leisure activities of adults with a psychotic disorder, a neurotic disorder, and no known psychiatric disorder, Great Britain, 1993*

Leisure activities	Adults with a psychotic disorder	Adults with a neurotic disorder	Adults with no known psychiatric disorder
Out of the home	*Percentage participating in each activity*		
Visiting friends or relatives	70	73	76
Pubs, restaurants	56	61	70
Shopping	56	66	68
Going for a walk, walking the dog	42	49	54
Sports as a participant	32	36	50
Cinema, theatre, concerts	43	38	46
Library	22	21	21
Clubs, organisations	28	15	20
Sports as a spectator	20	14	20
Night clubs, discos	28	16	18
Church	19	13	15
Classes or lectures	11	9	10
Bingo, amusement arcades	8	7	7
Bookmakers, betting and gambling	8	4	5
Political activities	1	2	1
In and around the home	*Percentage participating in each activity*		
TV/radio	80	87	91
Reading books/newspapers	56	66	71
Listening to music	73	67	67
Entertaining friends and relatives	48	51	56
Gardening	30	37	46
Writing letters/telephoning	33	38	36
Hobbies	48	35	34
Games	35	26	31
DIY/car maintenance	19	19	28
Base	*44*	*1557*	*8184*

Source: OPCS/ONS

Tables 4.7 and 4.8 provide further information about the economic activity, income and receipt of state benefits among those found to have neurotic or psychotic disorder. Comparisons with the adult general population are based on the OPCS Surveys of Psychiatric Morbidity or on the General Household or Omnibus Surveys carried out in 1993. Table 4.9 shows the level of participation in social activities. Tables 4.10 and 4.11 show the level of economic activity and the financial situation of adults with suicidal thoughts, compared with those who have neurotic disorders and with the general population.

This work provides for the first time a solid foundation of information about the extent of mental health problems in Great Britain. It is hoped that the survey will be repeated, perhaps at five-yearly intervals, to assess the impact of services. A further, more detailed study of information about those living in specialist residential facilities for people with mental health problems is in the planning stage. Other epidemiological work has identified significant psychiatric morbidity in other sub-groups of the population.

Table 4.10: *Economic activity of adults with suicidal thoughts compared with those with a neurotic disorder and those with no known psychiatric disorder, Great Britain, 1993*

	Adults with suicidal thoughts	Adults with a neurotic disorder	Adults with no known psychiatric disorder
	%	%	%
Working	27	56	71
Looking for work	17	11	7
Intending to look, temporarily sick	8	2	2
Permanently unable to work	16	12	2
Retired	2	2	4
Full time education	13	4	4
Keeping house	15	13	10
Other	2	1	1
Base	*80*	*1557*	*8184*

Source: OPCS/ONS

Table 4.11: *Financial situation of adults with suicidal thoughts compared with those with a neurotic disorder and with the general population, Great Britain, 1993*

	Adults with suicidal thoughts	Adults with a neurotic disorder	All adults surveyed in 1993 for the GHS/Omnibus Surveys[*]
State benefits	*Percentage receiving each State benefit*		
Income support	40	19	10
Invalidity pension, benefit or allowance	14	9	2
Sickness benefit	8	3	0
Disability living allowance	3	2	2
Attendance allowance	4	1	-
Base	*80*	*1557*	*13744*
Personal income	*Mid-point of income band*		
Median, weekly gross income	£70	£90	£150
Base	*80*	*1557*	*18760*

[*] State benefits data from GHS; income data from Omnibus survey.

Source: OPCS/ONS

Elderly people

The major mental health problems for older people are the dementias, which affect 5% of people aged over 65 years, and major depression, which also affects approximately 5%. The dementias include Alzheimer's disease, vascular dementia and Lewy body dementia, all of which show an increase in prevalence with increasing age; because of the ageing population, the current number of some 600,000 people with dementia in Great Britain may increase to about 800,000 by the year 2000, and one-third of these are likely to be severely affected.

Children and adolescents

Wallace and colleagues[10] define mental health problems in children and adolescents as "a disturbance of function in one area of relationships, mood, behaviour or development of sufficient severity to require professional intervention". The commonest functional disorders are emotional and conduct disorders, each with estimated prevalence rates of 5-10%. Between 1-3% of children have symptoms of depression. Substance misuse is a growing problem in adolescents; some 16% of 16-year-olds may regularly use solvents or other substances, with almost twice this number taking alcohol at least weekly from the early teenage years.

People with learning disabilities

Around 2% of the population have an identified learning disability, whilst about 0.3-0.4% have severe learning disabilities. The life expectancy of people with learning disabilities has improved during this century; children who might have died in infancy now survive to adulthood and adults live longer, which has increased the prevalence of people with profound or multiple handicaps and higher levels of dependency[11]. People with learning disabilities have an increased incidence of epilepsy, autism, cerebral palsy, communication disorders and impairments of vision and hearing, and are also at greater risk of a wide range of physical and mental health problems. *The Health of the Nation: a strategy for people with learning disabilities*[11] discusses many of these associated disorders, as well as issues for health promotion and health surveillance.

Ethnic minorities

Patterns of mental illnesses in African-Caribbean people indicate a high incidence of schizophrenia, which may be 3-6 times that of the indigenous population[12], although later studies[13] suggest regression towards the general population mean. In a more recent study[14], the prognosis of schizophrenia over four years of follow-up was better among people of African-Caribbean origin than in their white counterparts, although the former are more likely to be admitted under a section of the Mental Health Act 1983[15] and are more likely to be admitted to secure units[16]. Mental illness among people of Asian origin has been less extensively studied, but King and colleagues[13] found a higher incidence of schizophrenia in all ethnic minority groups, including Asian people, than in the indigenous population.

The Government has commissioned a large study through the Policy Studies Institute to examine mental health and patterns of service utilisation among people from ethnic minorities. This is the first study of its kind and should provide valuable information that will influence the future direction of research and service development for ethnic minorities. Ethnic monitoring of National Health Service (NHS) inpatients was introduced from 1 April 1995.

Suicide

The epidemiology of suicide in England has been described in a series of recent collaborative studies with the OPCS[17,18,19]. In England, suicide and undetermined deaths account for approximately 1% of all deaths (5,255 suicides and undetermined deaths in 1995), which represent 5% of all working days lost through death before the age of 65 years. It is the most common cause of death in 15-34-year-old males and females. Rates of suicide are four times higher among men than women (and three times higher among men for suicides and undetermined deaths), and this difference is increasing. Although motherhood does not protect against depression, mothers of young children are less likely to commit suicide. However, rates of suicide among immigrant populations are

Figure 4.4: *Standardised mortality rates* for suicide and undetermined injury, by age, England, 1970-95†*

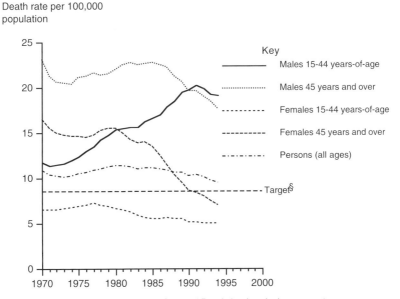

* Rates are calculated by use of the European Standard Population (to take into account differences in age structure) with a 3-year average plotted against middle year of average.
† Data for 1979 to 1995 excludes Inquest-adjourned cases (ICD E988.8). OPCS/ONS have recoded data for 1993 to 1995 on a comparable basis to those for 1992 and earlier years.
§ Target of 15% reduction for persons (all ages) from 1990 rate by year 2000.

Source: OPCS/ONS (ICD E950-E959, E980-E989 less E988.8)

107

higher among females (especially young Asian women who have rates six times higher than their white counterparts) than males[16]. Suicide rates are higher in individuals from social class V and among unemployed people, although under 10% of all those who commit suicide are unemployed. Severe mental disorder and alcohol abuse have a marked effect on lifetime suicide rates - which are estimated at 10% in schizophrenia, 15% in affective disorders and 15% in alcohol dependence[18]. Inhalation of car exhaust fumes is the means used in one-third of male suicides; self-poisoning has declined with reduced prescription for barbiturates, but still accounts for two-thirds of suicides among women, paracetamol being commonly used. Figure 4.4 shows standardised mortality rates for suicide and undetermined injury, by age and sex.

(ii)   Mental disorders in primary care

A recent World Health Organization (WHO) international collaborative study of mental health in primary care showed that well-defined psychological problems are common in all primary care settings (about 24% of all consultations)[20]. This finding is borne out by local English studies[21]. Although psychological disorders are common among people consulting in primary care, only around 5% volunteer psychological problems as the main reason for the visit - others tend to cite physical complaints. Family doctors only tend to assign a psychiatric diagnosis to about half of those who present with mental health problems. The research unit of the Royal College of General Practitioners (RCGP) has co-ordinated a survey of consultations with GPs in about 100 volunteer practices in decennial Census years since 1951. The fourth such survey indicates that mental health problems, as diagnosed by the GP, are the second most common reason for consultation[22].

(iii)   Information about specialist mental health services

Statistics about the activity of specialist mental health services in the NHS have been collected by DH for many years[23] to support policy development, strategic planning, the security and allocation of resources, and performance management. The current framework of information about episodes of admission and overall numbers of patient contacts was devised in the early 1980s and addressed only the information needs of management; data on the various components of each patient's care cannot be linked and thus the overall patterns of care given cannot be read directly. In view of developments in the approach to the management of people with chronic and severe mental disorders living in the community, and the need to collect information to monitor Health of the Nation targets[1], the Department is considering a revision of the framework for national mental health statistics to produce a system which reflects the complex multidisciplinary care arranged for such patients, including that provided outwith the NHS, and which is useful to clinical staff for clinical purposes. Care programme reviews form the key data capture point, and the data set would essentially comprise the framework of a current case summary with details of the patient, his or her problems and legal status, the care received since the last review and the current care plan[24]. A survey of all health authorities and providers of mental health care has shown widespread support for the approach[25], which is being tested in nine centres. Issues of confidentiality and data security will be critical. Guidance on these and related issues has recently been issued[26] and will be covered in *The protection and use of patient information*, to be issued to the NHS in early 1996.

(iv)   *Measuring mental health outcomes*

A key feature of the new mental health Data Set will be the Health of the Nation Outcome Scale (HoNOS)[27]. This twelve-item checklist has been developed for the Department by the Research Unit of the Royal College of Psychiatrists (RCPsych). In extensive field trials, the scale has been shown to have excellent inter-rater reliability and to show changes over time which closely reflect the clinical impression of the patient's progress. Two similar scales - one for use in child and adolescent mental health care and the other to improve the sensitivity of the present scale in assessing mental health problems in elderly people - are under development. The HoNOS scale will provide a detailed routine measure of progress towards the first target in the mental health key area of the Health of the Nation strategy[1].

(v)   *Confidential Inquiry into Homicides and Suicides by Mentally Ill People*

Two Health of the Nation targets[1] relate to suicides. A Confidential Inquiry into Homicides and Suicides by Mentally Ill People was established in 1992 and the first of two reports appeared[28,29]. The reports identify 39 cases of homicide (between July 1992 and March 1995) and 240 suicides; the inquiry has provided invaluable detailed insights into the events leading to such outcomes and the reports stress the need for:

— clarity of responsibilities, multidisciplinary co-operation and communication;

— treatment compliance;

— risk assessment skills;

— adequate staff numbers;

— audit programmes to maintain clinical skills;

— awareness of the quality of the patient's living environment;

— integration between voluntary and statutory sector service; *and*

— attention to the risk associated with changes in care regimens.

(vi)   *Research and development in mental health*

The Department's Research and Development (R&D) Directorate oversees two complementary research programmes which include mental health initiatives. The Policy Research Programme mental health initiative covers general mental health policy, and mentally disordered offenders, and projects in this programme will look at: mentally disordered offenders; suicides; mental health of ethnic minorities; various aspects of good care in the community; cognitive decline in elderly people; and the evaluation of administrative arrangements such as review tribunals and the introduction of supervision registers. Previously commissioned research on child and adolescent mental health includes parent training to cope with children with conduct disorders; deliberate self-harm in young people; detection of psychiatric disorder among adolescents attending GPs; and the development of culturally appropriate child and adolescent mental health services.

The first programme developed under the NHS R&D programme, initiated by the Central Research and Development Committee (CRDC), was for mental health, supported by an expert group chaired by Professor David Goldberg which identified five areas of national priority. These were taken forward by DH and the Medical Research Council (MRC), with £5 million made available centrally for such research. Regions were encouraged to commission and fund work in another 25 important areas in a programme co-ordinated and managed by Northern and Yorkshire Region. The top priorities cover: quality of life in residential care for elderly, mentally ill people; community care for severely mentally ill people; training packages for use in primary care and the community; mental health of the NHS workforce; and methodologies to establish the mental health needs of a particular population.

One of the reasons for the neglect and stigmatisation of mentally ill people has been that mental illness was poorly understood - but now this is changing, with exciting advances, such as in the impact of genetics on psychiatry and the collaboration between cognitive psychology and neuroimaging.

The delineation of the genetic contribution to psychiatric disorders such as autism, once thought to be the consequence of poor parenting, is a particularly striking example. This process also throws light on environmental influences on mental illness: genetic studies provide evidence for the existence of environmental influence and for the measurement of the variance accounted for by genetics, non-shared environment and shared environment. Social variables such as parental warmth, social support and life events may be partially subject to genetic influences, and common mental disorders are the result of interaction between multiple genetic and multiple environmental influences.

Recent advances in functional neuroimaging make it possible to observe directly brain function in vivo, and to observe the changes in blood-flow in small regions of the brain as specific processes are activated. The better understanding such techniques will provide for the working of the brain will greatly enhance our understanding of the mind.

(vii)   Public information strategy

The Government has also set up a three-year public information strategy to influence public attitudes to mental health services. This aims to increase understanding, reduce stigma and help users to understand both their rights and responsibilities. Since 1993, DH has spent £1 million on a public information campaign, with the aim of raising awareness and combating stigma; in 1996/97, £600,000 will be devoted to this work.

In addition to publishing specific mental health booklets[30,31,32,33,34,35,36,37], the Department is continuing to fund the work of the Health Education Authority (HEA), which is undertaking mental health promotion work focused on the World Mental Health Day in October 1996. This national campaign is facilitating local events across the country, particularly targeted on young people who are a key group to influence to achieve a real long-term change in public attitudes towards all mental illnesses. Overall, the Department will spend over £900,000 on mental health promotion and public information in 1996/97.

A new national Mental Health Awards scheme with three award categories to reward innovation and management in mental health services, focusing on effective working partnerships between different agencies, user-led services, and imaginative solutions for 'out-of-hours' services will be launched in 1996. The Department has also sponsored or been represented at conferences and events at which Health of the Nation messages[1] have been publicised, and has commissioned in each of the last three years a survey of public attitudes towards mental illness and mentally ill people. DH also supported the BBC Social Action series on mental health in Spring, 1995, and sponsored production of a Mental Health Directory to give details of local and national sources of help and information.

References

1. Department of Health. *The Health of the Nation: a strategy for health in England.* London: HMSO, 1992 (Cm. 1986).
2. Meltzer H, Gill B, Petticrew M, Hinds K. *The prevalence of psychiatric morbidity among adults living in private households.* London: HMSO, 1995 (OPCS Surveys of Psychiatric Morbidity in Great Britain: report 1).
3. Meltzer H, Gill B, Petticrew M, Hinds K. *Physical complaints, service use and treatment of adults with psychiatric disorders.* London: HMSO, 1995 (OPCS Surveys of Psychiatric Morbidity in Great Britain: report 2).
4. Meltzer H, Gill B, Petticrew M, Hinds K. *Economic activity and social functioning of adults with psychiatric disorders.* London: HMSO, 1995 (OPCS Surveys of Psychiatric Morbidity in Great Britain: report 3).
5. Meltzer H, Gill B, Petticrew M, Hinds K. *The prevalence of psychiatric morbidity among adults living in institutions.* London: HMSO (in press) (OPCS Surveys of Psychiatric Morbidity in Great Britain: report 4).
6. Meltzer H, Gill B, Petticrew M, Hinds K. *Physical complaints, service use and treatment of residents with psychiatric disorders.* London: HMSO (in press) (OPCS Surveys of Psychiatric Morbidity in Great Britain: report 5).
7. Meltzer H, Gill B, Petticrew M, Hinds K. *The economic activity and social functioning of residents with psychiatric disorders.* London: HMSO (in press) (OPCS Surveys of Psychiatric Morbidity in Great Britain: report 6).
8. Meltzer H, Gill B, Petticrew M, Hinds K. *Psychiatric morbidity among homeless people.* London: HMSO (in press) (OPCS Surveys of Psychiatric Morbidity in Great Britain: report 7).
9. Foster K, Meltzer H, Gill B, Petticrew M, Hinds K. *Adults with a psychotic disorder: living in the community.* London: HMSO (in press) (OPCS Surveys of Psychiatric Morbidity in Great Britain: report 8).
10. Wallace SA, Crown J, Cox A, Berger M. *Health care needs assessment: child and adolescent mental health.* Oxford: Radcliffe Medical (in press).

11. Department of Health. *The Health of the Nation: a strategy for people with learning disabilities.* London: HMSO, 1995.
12. Harrison G, Owen D, Holton A, Neilson D, Boot D. A prospective study of severe mental disorder in Afro-Caribbean patients. *Psychol Med* 1988; **18**: 643-57.
13. King M, Coker E, Leavey G, Hoare A, Johnson-Sabine E. Incidence of psychotic illness in London: a comparison of ethnic groups. *BMJ* 1994; **309**: 1115-9.
14. McKenzie K, van Os J, Fahy T et al. Psychosis with good prognosis in Afro-Caribbean people now living in the United Kingdom. *BMJ* 1995; **311**: 1325-7.
15. *The Mental Health Act 1983.* London: HMSO, 1983.
16. Raleigh S, Bulusu L, Balarajan R. Suicides among immigrants from the Indian sub-continent. *Br J Psychiatry* 1990; **156**: 46-50.
17. Charlton J, Kelly S, Dunnell K, Evans, Jenkins R, Wallis R. Trends in suicide deaths in England and Wales. *Population Trends* 1992; **69**: 10-6.
18. Charlton J, Kelly S, Dunnell K, Evans B, Jenkins R. Trends in factors associated with suicide deaths. *Population Trends* 1993; **71**: 34-42.
19. Charlton J, Kelly S, Jenkins R. Suicide deaths and occupations. *Population Trends* 1993; **73**: 42-8.
20. Sartorius N, Ustun T, Costa E Silva J et al. An international study of psychological problems in primary care: preliminary report from the WHO collaborative project on psychological problems in general health care. *Arch Gen Psychiatry* 1993; **50**: 819-24.
21. Goldberg D, Huxley P. *Common mental disorders: a biosocial model.* London: Routledge, 1992.
22. McCormick A, Fleming D, Charlton J. *Morbidity statistics from general practice: fourth national study: 1991-1992.* London: HMSO, 1995 (Series MB5 no. 3).
23. Department of Health. *Health and personal social services statistics for England.* London: HMSO, 1995.
24. Glover G. Mental health informatics and the rhythm of community care. *BMJ* 1995; **311**: 1038-9.
25. Dewhurst R. *Mental health minimum data set pilot: surveys of user views and provider systems.* London: Secta Consulting (in press).
26. Department of Health. *Building bridges.* London: Department of Health, 1995.
27. Department of Health. HoNOS: a psychiatric thermometer. *CMO's Update* 1994; **7**: 7.
28. Confidential Inquiry into Homicides and Suicides by Mentally Ill People. *A preliminary report on homicides.* London: Royal College of Psychiatrists, 1994.
29. Steering Committee of the Confidential Inquiry into Homicides and Suicides by Mentally Ill People. *Report of the Confidential Inquiry into Homicides and Suicides by Mentally Ill People.* London: Royal College of Psychiatrists (in press).
30. Department of Health. *Mental illness: what does it mean?* London: Department of Health, 1993.
31. Department of Health. *Mental illness: what you can do about it.* London: Department of Health, 1994.
32. Department of Health. *Mental illness: a guide to mental health in the workplace.* London: Department of Health, 1993.
33. Department of Health. *Mental illness: mental health and older people.* London: Department of Health, 1994.
34. Department of Health. *Mental illness: can children and young people have mental health problems?* London: Department of Health, 1994.
35. Department of Health. *Mental illness: sometimes I think I can't go on anymore.* London: Department of Health, 1993.
36. Department of Health. *Down on the farm? Coping with depression in rural areas: a farmer's guide.* London: Department of Health, 1995.
37. Department of Health. *Mental health: towards a better understanding.* London: Department of Health, 1995.

(c)   Development of services for mental health care

The goals for the DH mental health strategy are to: promote mental health, prevent mental illness, improve health and social functioning, and reduce mortality. These goals are embraced in the Health of the Nation targets for mental illness[1].

The *Mental illness key area handbook*[2] outlines a number of crucial aims of the strategy including:

— to augment local comprehensive secondary care services to ensure adequate facilities for people with severe mental illness;

— to support primary care services to ensure effective management of people suffering from more common, less severe forms of mental disorder;

— to ensure good physical and dental care for people with mental disorders;

— to develop good practice through dissemination of research and information and encouragement of local clinical practice guidelines;

— to improve inter-agency working between health and social services, housing, the police, probation services and the criminal justice system, and non-statutory agencies;

— to emphasise the need for adequate housing for vulnerable individuals living in the community;

— to reduce stigmatisation of people with mental disorders through public education; *and*

— to promote mental health.

Specific resources are available to develop the spectrum of services needed to ensure that high quality care and treatment is provided to all people with mental health problems. The Mental Illness Specific Grant has made an important contribution to the improvement of the health and social care of individuals with severe mental disorders; over 1,200 projects have been funded since it was introduced in 1988. In 1996, the Mental Health Challenge Fund will also be available and will particularly encourage health authorities to devote more money towards specific improvements in mental health services.

(i) *Children and adolescents*

The Department has commissioned several research projects into child and adolescent mental health services (CAMHS). A study on such services throughout England[3] indicated that the "matching of provision to local needs had hardly begun" and helped to focus three other initiatives designed to assist purchasers and providers of care in the development of comprehensive CAMHS.

The DH *Handbook on child and adolescent mental health*[4], launched in March, was followed by the Health Advisory Service's review *Together we stand*[5]

In November, a guide to the assessment of need in child and adolescent mental health was made available[6]; this guidance has been backed by a performance management programme to assist purchasers in service developments and to meet the objectives in the NHS *Priorities and planning guidance[7]*.

The mental health of children and young people is not the concern of the NHS alone. All involved in the care of the young have a part to play; the guidance views services in flexible and dynamic tiers, reflecting the setting in which children and families may receive help, the severity of their problems and the nature of any intervention required.

Although research findings indicate a significant prevalence of such problems in young people, relatively few children are recognised by their GP to have mental health problems; only about 10% of children who have such problems are referred to specialist services[8]. Several initiatives involving GPs and health visitors are intended to increase awareness and knowledge of such challenges in the primary care setting. Secondary care services should be multidisciplinary and focus on the assessment and treatment of children with more complex problems, with well-established co-ordination and liaison with all child agencies. Tertiary level services offer specialist help to children from more than one district; inpatient services for adolescents are contracted on this basis, but there are also specialist outpatient assessment and treatment services.

Some of the greatest challenges for planning and co-ordinating services lie at the interfaces of specialist CAMHS with social services, the criminal justice system, acute paediatric care and community child health care, and it is important for all agencies to share priorities - and the main priority is the care and welfare of children, young people and their families.

(ii)   Adults with mental health problems

A wide range of mental disorders is seen in primary care settings. A recent survey[9] indicated that one-quarter of consecutive attenders at GP surgeries had at least one, and 14% had at least two, mental ill-health diagnoses. The commonest was depression (17%), followed by anxiety states and panic disorder (11% each), chronic fatigue (10%) and alcohol problems (4%). Family doctors assign mental ill-health diagnoses to about half of those people at risk, only about 10% of whom are seen and treated by specialised mental illness services. The White Paper *Caring for people[10]* promised an examination of primary mental health care to see what practical steps could be taken to improve it. The Department sponsored a series of conferences - 'Counselling in general practice'[11] 'Prevention of depression and anxiety: the role of the primary care team'[12], 'Primary care of schizophrenia'[13] and 'Mental health promotion and prevention of mental illness in primary care'[14] - which brought together experts to present the main issues, debate future strategies and disseminate ideas about good practice. In parallel with these conferences, DH funded projects from the

114

National Development Fund for new initiatives in primary care to provide a basis for educational programmes[15].

Since 1992, the RCGP and the RCPsych have co-operated in a 'Defeat depression' campaign: videotapes on depression have been prepared and distributed to teachers of GPs, a book on depression has been sent to all members of the RCGP[16], and every GP has been sent guidelines on the treatment of depression[17]. The effectiveness of the campaign is being evaluated. DH has partly funded a senior mental health educational Fellow at the RCGP since 1992 to take a national lead on continuing medical education in mental health for GPs and the primary care team, and to develop training packages and establish a regional network of trainers who have developed learner-centred, practice-based methods of training. The RCGP unit for mental health education in primary care is developing teacher training, a series of study days for primary care team members, and practice-based training.

DH has also funded a national mental health trainer, through the Mental Health Foundation, to the nurse facilitator project, who is based in the RCGP unit for mental health education to provide support to and to train primary care facilitators in mental health. The Department has also funded a national mental health audit Fellow to work in the unit to provide a comprehensive yet 'practice-friendly' audit package that covers the main mental health problems seen in primary care.

(iii)   *Adults with severe mental illness*

During the 19th Century and early part of the 20th Century, large asylums were built in England in rural settings on the edge of towns and cities. They were seen at the time as a great humanitarian step towards solving the problems of people with severe mental illness - delivering care, treatment, food, shelter and occupational activities. However, until the 1940s, admissions to these large institutions exceeded discharges, leading to the accumulation of large numbers of long-stay residents; such patients led an existence notable for its social poverty and consequent harm to the social functioning of patients, as shown by research on the effects of institutionalisation. The Mental Health Act 1959[18] ensured that only people whose mental disorder was so severe that treatment in hospital was necessary in the interest of the patient's health and safety, or for the protection of others, were detained in hospital. In 1961, the then Minister for Health announced a reprovision programme to accompany the asylum closure programme, noting the requirement for "an almost unlimited range of gradation between the complete independence of full mental and physical health and the almost complete dependence of those whose need for care and attention is little short of that which only a hospital can provide". In 1975, the Government published a White Paper *Better services for the mentally ill*[19], which set out the policy framework for service development; it proposed comprehensive local care, including small acute units, residential accommodation and community services.

In August 1995, the Minister for Health asked NHS regional directors to review the progress made in their regions towards the delivery of modern and effective mental health services. Although the results of that review, to be published in February 1996, showed that every health authority now has a strategic plan for fully comprehensive local services, many still had progress to make towards achieving them. These will continue to be monitored until fully implemented. The Government is committed to deliver not simply care in the community, but the full spectrum of care required for a comprehensive local modern mental health service, where people are looked after as close to home as is compatible with the health and safety of themselves and the public. This spectrum includes inpatient beds, new long-stay 24-hour nursed care, supported housing, work, occupational rehabilitation, education, vocational training and leisure activities[20]. This overall spectrum of care is provided and funded by a number of different organisations, and requires careful consideration by commissioners and providers of health care, bearing in mind the needs of each individual client.

Many people with severe mental illness may need support and treatment for the rest of their lives. Hospital admission may be needed from time to time, although in some instances crisis services (such as teams able to provide care at home for short periods of time or a 'safe house' to offer short-term care) may be a better alternative. A small number of people, with the most complex and challenging problems, require longer term 24-hour nursed care[21]; in the absence of such provision, these individuals take up acute beds, with the result that many patients needing urgent but brief admissions for relapse are unable to obtain a local bed, resulting in costly extra-contractual referrals to other districts or to the private sector.

The care programme approach (CPA)[22] was introduced in 1991 to ensure: services assess needs for health and social care; a package of care is assembled to meet those needs, drawn up in agreement with the multidisciplinary health team, social services, GPs, user and carers; a key worker is appointed to keep close contact with the patient; and that regular review and monitoring of the patient's needs and progress, and of the delivery of care, takes place. The CPA is tiered, so that patients with the greatest needs receive the most comprehensive package of care. Supervision registers[23] were introduced to identify patients who are at significant risk of suicide, serious harm to others or serious self-neglect. They are a flexible and temporary priority listing of those on the CPA who are considered most at risk. As well as identifying who provides input from the secondary services, the primary care team's involvement and knowledge of the patient and their family is taken account of in the CPA. The primary care team will then be able to communicate change in the clinical condition through the key worker to the appropriate professional. The role of the practice nurse may also be developed to include administration of depot neuroleptic medication and monitoring of clinical progress[24]. People with severe mental illness need access to good quality physical and dental health care and health promotion, which will be provided by the primary care medical and dental services.

Last year, DH undertook to review the provision and purchasing of psychotherapies as part of its policy to promote clinically effective, cost-effective care and evidence-based practice. The review, which is now almost complete, will examine research in detail and will make recommendations on how to interpret research on effectiveness in the talking therapies, and identify implications for purchasers, practitioners, trainers and the public. The report will be published during 1996.

Primary/secondary care interface

Secondary care services should give priority to the treatment of people with severe mental illness; some secondary care service activity is devoted to the management of commoner and less complicated disorders, possibly as a reflection of less primary mental health care activity particularly in some inner-city areas. Secondary services must achieve a careful balance between facilitating primary mental health care by improving routes of communication and access for more difficult mental health problems, particularly when these pose a high level of risk to the patient or others, and supporting primary health care staff in dealing with the most common and more manageable problems themselves.

Co-morbidity

There are high levels of co-morbidity between mental and physical ill-health. When medical and surgical inpatients are screened for mental health problems, alcohol and drug misuse, many otherwise unrecognised cases are observed. A growing number of district general hospitals now include in their clinical resources a consultant liaison psychiatrist and medical psychologists. The complexity of secondary care psychiatric services, which will have to deal with such cases following discharge from a medical or surgical bed, also demands the close involvement of psychiatry professionals in the work on general wards and accident and emergency departments.

Homeless mentally ill initiative

This was announced in July 1990 in response to concerns about the health and safety of homeless mentally ill people on the streets of London. Some £20 million have now been spent on this initiative, which offers multidisciplinary community mental health outreach to identify clients who have lost contact with health services, to establish their needs, and to give them access to rehabilitation hostel places and, through housing corporations, more permanent accommodation.

Eating disorders

Most health districts provide either local specialised treatment in a psychiatric inpatient unit for patients with eating disorders or contract out to a specialised unit elsewhere. These patients require specialised treatment, not only because of the high mortality associated with the more severe forms of eating disorder, but also because of the exceptional demands made on staff caring for people with such problems.

Perinatal mental health

There is a steep rise in the incidence of severe mental illness in women following childbirth. The risk of admission with psychosis in the 30 days following childbirth is increased by a factor of 21, and the risk of developing major depressive illness is increased three-fold. Postnatal depression occurs in 10-15% of women having a baby; it is the most common of all serious complications (physical or psychological) of the puerperium[25]. DH and the RCPsych have set up a joint working party to develop guidelines for purchasers and providers of health care on the development of perinatal mental health services; it is due to report in Autumn, 1996.

Mental health of prisoners

There is a high prevalence of mental disorder among convicted and remand prisoners alike. Over one-third of male convicted prisoners have a mental disorder, 23% misuse substances and 2% have psychosis - similar to the findings of a survey some 20 years before[26,27]. Mental disorder is even commoner in remand prisoners; two-thirds of males and 77% of females have at least one diagnosis, most commonly substance misuse (39% of men and 42% of women). Prisoners who meet the criteria for admission under the Mental Health Act 1983[28] need transfer to health service care; such transfers have increased seven-fold between 1981 and 1994.

Mentally disordered offenders

Challenges in the care of mentally disordered offenders are discussed in the Introduction (see page 5).

Mental health legislation

The Mental Health Act 1983[28] allows for the detention in hospital of people with a mental disorder of a nature or degree which makes medical treatment in hospital appropriate, if this is necessary for the health or safety of the patient or the protection of others. Detained patients may be treated without consent in specified circumstances, but such treatment outside hospital is not permitted except in an emergency. The Mental Health (Patients in the Community) Act 1995[29] has introduced new legal powers to help to ensure that detained patients who are at special risk receive suitable care following discharge from hospital.

(iv) People with learning disabilities

In the years since the White Paper *Better services for the mentally handicapped*[30], care and support for people with learning disabilities has shifted towards an approach based on individual needs. In common with the rest of the population, people with learning disabilities have physical and emotional needs that will be provided by a normal and healthy lifestyle. The residents of hospitals have been moved to a wide range of community alternatives, with social services as the leading agency in their development. During 1994-95, the

Social Services Inspectorate (SSI) mounted an inspection of leisure and recreation facilities in day-care services[31]; a national development team has been commissioned to produce a handbook based on the experiences of hospital closure; and research was commissioned to evaluate various types of non-hospital accommodation and support.

Most people with a learning disability have additional needs for support due to their cognitive difficulties. Grants have been given to a number of independent organisations to explore approaches to deal with such vulnerability. People with learning disabilities should benefit from all the actions that are taken to improve the health of the whole population[32]. The 'Continuing the commitment' project for learning disability nursing[33] has identified a role for nurses in health surveillance and health promotion, and in developing the personal competence of service users.

The association between learning disability, other disabilities and health-related problems means that some people with learning disabilities have complex health and social care needs. Guidelines on health services for people with learning disabilities[34] state that commissioners of care should consider contracts for additional services for people with learning disabilities; there are also likely to be a few people with severe or profound disabilities and physical, sensory or psychiatric conditions who require long-term residential care. Some people with learning disabilities need treatment for psychiatric illness or behaviour disturbance. If it is not possible adequately to meet those needs within general psychiatric services, specialist assessment and treatment services will be needed in hospital or community settings. A number of different service models have been developed and evaluation of these is required. The Mansell report[34] emphasises that priority should be given to improve the capability of mainstream learning disability services to prevent problems arising in the first place; to manage them when they occur; and to implement sophisticated long-term arrangements for management, treatment and care. To facilitate the implementation of this report, a National Implementation Network was funded and an Advisory Group on Behavioural Disturbance and Mental Health Service Developments was established for two years.

(v)   Older people with mental health problems

GPs retain their roles as gatekeepers to specialist multidisciplinary old age psychiatry services, but with the implementation of the NHS and Community Care Act 1990[35] social services now purchase most continuing support for older people with mental health problems. The major mental health problems for older people are dementias and affective disorders; the diagnosis of both can be difficult in old age. Depressive illness is at least as treatable as in younger age-groups. An accurate diagnosis of dementia is important as a significant minority have treatable associated physical illnesses and knowledge of the diagnosis and prognosis is important for carers and to develop support packages to allow people to remain in a homely setting, often their own home, for as long as it is safe and prudent to do so. This may require organisation of a range of help from the statutory sector, including social care from social workers and home helps;

voluntary sector care including sitting services; and financial and other support: a small group of patients may require inpatient continuing care provided by the NHS. Specialist old-age psychiatry teams have an integrated approach to working across from the community, through day hospitals and into inpatient services, working closely with local and social services and with colleagues in geriatric medicine.

In 1994, Ministers asked DH to develop a strategy for elderly mentally ill people. Certain actions had already been implemented in isolation but, in future, work will be taken forward in a more co-ordinated manner - with liaison with non-statutory organisations; a Health Needs Assessment Review of dementia to assist purchasers of care; input to the 'Defeat depression' campaign; production of booklets for the general public (eg, *Mental health and older people*[36]) and for purchasers (eg, *Patient perception series: dementia*[37]); and, as part of the GP contract, an annual health check is offered to each patient aged 75 years and over. The SSI is also developing three projects, reporting in 1996, on multidisciplinary assessments to identify the needs of people with dementia; on elderly mentally infirm people living alone, to identify the issues in providing services; and a national inspection of services to develop standards.

References

1. Department of Health. *The Health of the Nation: a strategy for health in England.* London: HMSO, 1992 (Cm. 1986).
2. Department of Health. *Mental illness key area handbook, 2nd edn.* London: HMSO, 1994.
3. Kurtz Z, Thornes R, Wolkind S. *Services for the mental health of children and young people in England: a national review.* London: Maudsley Hospital and South Thames (West) Regional Health Authority, 1994.
4. Department of Health, Social Services Inspectorate, Department for Education. *A handbook on child and adolescent mental health.* London: HMSO, 1995.
5. Health Advisory Service. *Child and adolescent mental health services: together we stand: the commissioning role and management of child and adolescent mental health services.* London: HMSO, 1995.
6. Wallace SA, Crown JM, Cox AD, Berger M. *Health care needs assessment: child and adolescent mental health.* In: Stevens A, Raftery J, eds. *Health care needs assessment: series 2.* Oxford: Radcliffe Medical (in press).
7. Department of Health. *Priorities and planning guidance for the NHS: 1996/97.* Wetherby (West Yorkshire): Department of Health, 1995.
8. Rutter M, Tizard J, Whitmore K. *Education, health and behaviour.* London: Longman, 1970.
9. Sartorius N, Ustun T, Costa E Silva J. An international study of psychological problems in primary care. *Arch Gen Psychiatry*, 1993; **50**: 819-24.
10. Department of Health. *Caring for people: community care in the next decade and beyond.* London: HMSO, 1989 (Cm. 849).
11. Corney R, Jenkins R. *Counselling in general practice.* London: Routledge, 1992.
12. Jenkins R, Newton J, Young R. *The prevention of depression and anxiety.* London: HMSO, 1992.
13. Jenkins R, Field V, Young R. *The primary care of schizophrenia: a conference organised by R&D for Psychiatry and the Department of Health.* London: HMSO, 1992.
14. Jenkins R, Ustun T. *Mental health promotion and prevention.* London: HMSO (in press).
15. Jenkins R. Developments in the primary care of mental illness: a forward look. *Int Rev Psychiatry* 1992; **4**: 237-42.
16. Wright A. *Depression: recognition and management in general practice.* London: Royal College of General Practitioners, 1993.
17. Department of Health. *Defeat depression: recognition and management of depression in general practice.* London: Department of Health, 1993.

18. *The Mental Health Act 1959*. London: HMSO, 1959.
19. Department of Health and Social Security. *Better services for the mentally ill*. London: HMSO, 1975 (Cm. 6233).
20. Department of Health. *The spectrum of care: local services for people with mental disorders*. Wetherby (West Yorkshire): Department of Health (in press).
21. NHS Executive. *24-hour nursed care for people with severe and enduring mental illness*. Wetherby (West Yorkshire): Department of Health (in press).
22. Department of Health. *Caring for people: the care programme approach for people with a mental illness referred to the specialist psychiatric services*. London: Department of Health, 1990 (Health Circular: HC(90)23).
23. NHS Management Executive. *Introduction of supervision registers for mentally ill people from 1 April 1994*. Leeds: Department of Health, 1994 (Health Service Guidelines: HSG(94)5).
24. Department of Health, Royal College of Nursing. *Good practice in the administration of depot neuroleptics*. London: Department of Health, 1994.
25. Prettyman RJ, Friedman T. Care of women with puerperal psychiatric disorders in England and Wales. *BMJ* 1991; **302**: 1245-6.
26. Gunn J, Robertson G, Dell S, Wang C. *Psychiatric aspects of imprisonment*. London: Academic Press, 1978.
27. Gunn J, Maden A, Swinton S. Treatment needs of prisoners with psychiatric disorders. *BMJ* 1991; **303:** 338-41.
28. *The Mental Health Act 1983*. London: HMSO, 1983.
29. *The Mental Health (Patients in the Community) Act 1995*. London: HMSO, 1995.
30. Department of Health and Social Security. *Better services for the mentally handicapped*. London: HMSO, 1980.
31. Social Services Inspectorate. *Leisure and recreation facilities*. London: Social Services Inspectorate (in press).
32. Department of Health. *Health services for people with learning disabilities (mental handicap)*. Wetherby (West Yorkshire): Department of Health, 1992 (Health Service Guidelines HSG(92)42).
33. Kay B, Rose S, Turnbull J. *Continuing the commitment: the report of the Learning Disability Nursing Project*. London: Department of Health, 1995.
34. Department of Health. *Services for people with learning disabilities and challenging behaviour or mental health needs: report of a project group*. London: HMSO, 1993. Chair: Dr James Mansell.
35. *The NHS and Community Care Act 1990*. London: HMSO, 1990.
36. Department of Health. *Mental health and older people*. London: HMSO, 1994.
37. NHS Executive. *Patient perception series: dementia*. Leeds: Department of Health, 1994.

(d)   The way ahead

(i)   Mental health promotion

Primary prevention is intended to prevent the onset of mental disorder; secondary prevention to detect and treat mental disorder early; and tertiary prevention to maintain the health and social functioning of people with a diagnosed mental disorder[1].

Primary prevention

This includes strategies to reduce the occurrence of risk-factors and to improve the coping response triggered by stress factors. There are several different levels of intervention. Mental health education seeks to inform the general public about mental health problems and about available treatment and health promotion resources. Research indicates that people often have minimal knowledge about local mental health services. It is particularly important to reduce stigma, and schools and the media have a crucial role. Mental health education also aims to develop important competencies within at-risk groups and the general population to improve the capacity to cope with predictable life transitions and with less predictable stress. Parenting classes in schools and for young parents are important examples.

Secondary prevention

GPs, health visitors and others can be encouraged to look for mental disorders in high-risk groups such as postnatal women, children in families with a single parent, people with chronic physical or with terminal illness, people with a disability, carers and people who live alone. Early recognition of mental disorders is facilitated by longer consultation times and an open consulting style. Early treatment may prevent the development of chronic or secondary problems. Continuing treatment of depression for several months after symptom resolution may prevent relapse. The International Classification of Diseases (ICD)-10-based primary health care guidelines are designed to augment mental health assessment and management skills and to achieve earlier treatment.

Tertiary prevention

Effective treatment of people with persistent disorders, especially severe mental illness, will improve outcome. Addressing housing and social needs, as well as medical needs, may help to maintain social networks and lead to a better quality of life. Support or family therapy can reduce stress and also prevent relapse in individuals with disorders such as depression and schizophrenia.

(ii)   Clinical practice guidelines

Clinical practice guidelines (CPGs) were first developed in Australia in the early 1980s for the management of depression. The most highly developed CPG, also on depression, was devised in the USA[2]. Funding has now been provided to the RCPsych research unit to devise CPGs that are applicable in the UK. The unit has produced a detailed protocol for the development of guidelines and is collaborating closely with the Cochrane Review. Its first CPG, which deals with risk assessment and management, will be completed in 1996. The Royal College and the Department are working together to explore ways to implement CPGs through continuing medical education and through performance management of purchasing by local health authorities.

(iii)   Suicide prevention

Suicide prevention needs to: reduce access to means; increase public awareness; target high-risk groups; and develop primary and secondary care[3,4].

Evidence from the 1970s, when highly toxic coal gas was replaced by North Sea gas as a source of domestic fuel, indicates that, when access to a particular means of suicide is reduced, only a proportion of potential victims switch to another method. Restriction of access to commonly used means of suicide is therefore potentially an important public health measure. Analgesics (principally paracetamol) account for over 500 suicides and undetermined deaths annually (around 10% of the total), and are the most common means of suicide apart from car exhaust gases and hanging; options under consideration include limiting pack sizes or restricting sale to pharmacies. Certain antidepressants can be lethal if taken in sufficient quantities; options for restriction might include wider use of blister packs, and restriction of single supplies to 7 or 14 days at standard dosage to reduce the availability of potentially lethal quantities. Car exhaust gases are the single most common means of suicide, particularly among younger men, accounting for nearly 6,000 deaths during 1988-92; the progressive introduction of catalytic converters should reduce these deaths, and a further option may be to modify car exhausts to make it more difficult to attach a hose.

The vast majority of people who commit suicide are suffering at the time from a treatable mental disorder, often depression. Greater awareness of the problems of suicide and depression can encourage sufferers (or others, such as their family) to seek appropriate help. Groups who can be targeted include: professionals, such as teachers, probation officers, and prison staff, who work with groups of people who are at particularly high risk; primary health care workers, including GPs, health visitors and district nurses; and the general public. Messages include "get advice if someone talks of committing suicide, even if they don't want you to", and "understandable depression still needs treatment". DH's public information strategy has issued a booklet *Sometimes I think I can't go on any more* about suicide[5].

High-risk groups include: certain occupations (eg, veterinary surgeons, doctors, nurses, dentists and farmers); people with specific diagnoses, such as terminal illness and those in chronic pain; severely mentally ill people, particularly those with depression or with hallucinations that may lead to self-harm; relatives of people who have committed suicide; people with a history of suicide attempts or self-harm; drug and alcohol abusers; young people at risk such as those from broken homes, in care or with criminal records; people who are affected by bankruptcy or redundancy; and homeless people. Ministers have met with leaders of high-risk professional groups to discuss the development of suicide prevention strategies. Work is being sponsored at the University of Oxford to audit suicides in high-risk occupational groups, and local and national initiatives to tackle the problem of rural stress include a DH information booklet on depression and suicide targeted specifically at farmers[6].

Most people who commit suicide are suffering from a mental illness at the time, and a high proportion will have had recent contact with the health services (particularly their GP). Further developments in health services could be targeted on improving the detection and management of mental illness, such as: improved documentation and communication of self-harm histories; better GP training in the detection and management of depression; better detection and management of suicide risks in accident and emergency units; and improved risk assessment for severely mentally ill people. Supervision registers have been introduced to help local health services to identify mentally ill people who are at serious risk of suicide or self-harm, or of harming others. Implementation of the care programme approach should ensure that community-based mental health care addresses patients' properly assessed needs in a co-ordinated fashion. The NHS Executive has also published guidance on the assessment of self-harm cases in accident and emergency departments[7].

(iv)   *Ensuring a healthy workforce*

Studies of minor psychiatric morbidity in working populations indicate a high prevalence of between 27-37%[8]. Minor psychiatric disorder is a major determinant of sickness absence, and is the second most common cause of prolonged absence. Within the workplace, people suffering from mental health problems may work less effectively and their relationships with colleagues and customers may be impaired. The stigma that still attaches to mental health problems makes it difficult accurately to assess the total cost to industry, although current estimates place the annual cost at well over £3,700 million. As part of the Health of the Nation strategy[9], the Department has been working to increase employers' awareness of the issues and to encourage them to take appropriate action by sponsoring conferences and producing booklets for employers[8], and by commissioning training material to help business schools to train employers on how to deal with mental health problems. To ensure co-ordination of such strategies, DH convened the Mental Health at Work Inter-Agency Group, including representation from the Confederation of British Industry (CBI), the Trades Union Congress, the Health and Safety Executive (HSE), the Advisory Conciliation and Arbitration Service, the HEA, the Institute of Personnel Management, and the Small Business Federation.

A survey by the CBI and DH in 1991 showed that although 95% of responding employers thought that mental illness should be of concern to their organisation, only 12% had a company policy on mental health. The employers' survey was repeated in late 1995 and results will be available in 1996. DH issued its own policy on mental health in 1994 and has produced a number of booklets and resource packs[10,11]. Interim research reports on the mental health of the NHS workforce points to the importance of occupational health policies that address mental as well as physical health. In May 1995, the HSE issued guidance on workplace stress[12]; research indicates that harmful levels of stress can lead to psychological problems such as depression and anxiety[13]. The HSE guidance[12], which is targeted particularly at smaller employers, emphasises a preventive approach. The HSE has commissioned a further programme of research into this area. A senior occupational health Fellow has been funded to promote the education of occupational health staff about mental health both in private health care and in the NHS. In addition, DH has funded two part-time GP Fellows at the RCGP to increase awareness of stress among GPs and to promote sensible solutions.

(v)   *International links*

DH's mental health division maintains close collaboration with the World Health Organization (WHO) and with mental health policy-makers around the world. In

1995, it contributed to a number of WHO Task Forces on global action for improvement of mental health care, primary care of mental health, epidemiology for developing countries, systems for assessment of psychiatric care and a WHO/European Task Force on prevention. The division contributed consultancy to the English-speaking Caribbean on mental health services, members to an international panel to review Sweden's mental health services at the invitation of the Swedish Government, and workshops to the Ministries of Health in Victoria, South Australia and New South Wales in Australia, and to New Zealand. A number of countries are now making extensive use of the Health of the Nation[9] implementation strategy on mental illness, the key area handbook[11], the methodology for national surveys, and the Health of the Nation outcome scales[14].

DH also collaborated with WHO to produce an international conference in July 1995 on mental health promotion and primary prevention in primary care.

(vi) Mental health into the 21st Century

Mental health has long been regarded as a mysterious, enigmatic, difficult and even frightening topic to contemplate, touching as it does on the soul and the personality as well as the essential processes of thought, cognition and perception. Thus while we all prize our own mental health, people who have mental illness and those who devote their lives to working with them have at some times in the past been stigmatised, undervalued and under-resourced. Mental health should be valued as much as physical health, and health policies and initiatives in the workplace and schools, as well as in the NHS, ought to include a proper focus on mental health. The choice of mental illness as a key area in the Health of the Nation initiative[9], and as a priority in NHS priorities and planning guidance, are key steps to bring mental health to the forefront of medical practice. Mental health problems remain a leading cause of the public health burden of disease in this and all other countries around the world, and need to be vigorously tackled towards and beyond the targets set in the strategy for health[9] (see Table 4.12). A sound research base is essential: the Institute of Psychiatry in London is internationally acknowledged as a leading research institution for the impact of its research, and strong research teams in mental

Table 4.12: *Main targets for mental illness**

To improve significantly the health and social functioning of mentally ill people

To reduce the overall suicide rate by at least 15% by the year 2000 *(Baseline 1990)*

To reduce the suicide rate of severely mentally ill people by at least 33% by the year 2000 *(Baseline 1990)*

---

* The 1990 baseline for all mortality targets represents an average of three years centred around 1990.

health are also well developed elsewhere in the country. This research capacity must be nurtured and its continuing integration with health and social services for mental health encouraged, so that it continues to provide the bedrock for yet further progress.

References

1. Paykel ES, Jenkins R. *Prevention in psychiatry: report of the Special Committee on the Place of Prevention in Psychiatry.* London: Gaskell, 1994.
2. Depression Guideline Panel. *Depression in primary care: vol 2: treatment of major depression.* Upland (Pennsylvania), USA: Diane Publications, 1994.
3. Jenkins R, Griffiths S, Hawton K, Morgan G, Tylee A, Wylie I, eds. *The prevention of suicide.* London: HMSO, 1994.
4. Kingdon DG, Jenkins R. *Suicide prevention.* In: Phelan M, Thornicroft G, eds. *Emergency psychiatric services.* London: Routledge, 1995.
5. Department of Health. *Mental illness: sometimes I think I can't go on any more.* London: Department of Health, 1994.
6. Department of Health. *Down on the farm? Coping with depression in rural areas: a farmer's guide.* London: Department of Health, 1995.
7. NHS Executive. *Guidance on the assessment of self-harm cases in accident and emergency departments.* Leeds: Department of Health, 1995.
8. Jenkins R, Warman D. *Promoting mental health policies in the workplace.* London: HMSO, 1993.
9. Department of Health. *The Health of the Nation: a strategy for health in England.* London: HMSO, 1992 (Cm. 1986).
10. Department of Health. *ABC of mental health in the workplace: resource pack for employers.* London: Department of Health, 1995.
11. Department of Health. *Mental illness: key area handbook,* 2nd edn. London: HMSO, 1994.
12. Health and Safety Executive. *Stress at work: a guide for employers.* London: Health and Safety Executive, 1995.
13. Health and Safety Executive. *Stress research and stress management: putting theory to work.* London: Health and Safety Executive, 1993 (Contract Research Report no. 61/1993).
14. Department of Health. HoNOS: a psychiatric thermometer. *CMO's Update* 1994; **4:** 7.

CHAPTER 5

HEALTH CARE

(a)   Role and function of the National Health Service in England

(i)   Strategic purpose

The purpose of the National Health Service (NHS) is to secure through the resources available the greatest possible improvement to the physical and mental health of the people of England by: promoting health, preventing ill-health, diagnosing and treating disease and injury, and caring for those with long-term illness and disability who require the services of the NHS - a service available to all on the basis of clinical need, regardless of the ability to pay.

In seeking to achieve this purpose as a public service, the NHS aims to judge its results under three headings:

—   *equity;* by improving the health of the population as a whole and reducing variations in health status by targeting resources where needs are greatest;

—   *efficiency;* by providing patients with treatment and care that is both clinically effective and a good use of taxpayers' money; *and*

—   *responsiveness;* by meeting the needs of individual patients and ensuring that the NHS changes appropriately as those needs change, and as medical knowledge advances.

(ii)   Policies

The Health of the Nation White Paper[1] remains the central plank of Government policy for the NHS. It provides a strategic approach to enhance the overall health of the population, setting targets for improving health in five key areas and emphasising disease prevention and health promotion. Much progress has been achieved both in embedding the Health of the Nation initiative within the NHS and in pursuing its objectives across the community in partnership with other agencies, but much more remains to be done (see also page 90).

Three other Government policies remain of central importance to the strategic purpose of the NHS, and for obtaining the benefits of greater equity, efficiency and responsiveness.

The community care reforms as set out in *Caring for people*[2] aim to allow vulnerable people to live as independently as possible in their own homes or in a homely setting in the community. The emphasis is on releasing resources from institutional care to fund more flexible and appropriate care for patients within their local community. The development of community care remained a high priority during 1995. Guidance issued in February on NHS responsibilities for continuing health care[3] provided a framework for local policies and eligibility criteria for services, ranging from continuing inpatient care, rehabilitation, and palliative care to services in the community. Following consultation with interested parties, agreed eligibility criteria are to be put into operation from April 1996. Collaboration between health and local authorities in the commissioning of community care services, with the aim of better integration of services for users and carers, has been encouraged with guidance on joint commissioning[4] published in May.

The patient's charter[5] initiative aims to put patients first by the provision of services which meet clearly defined national and local standards and by responding to people's views and needs. From April, the guaranteed maximum waiting time for patients to be admitted to hospital for treatment was brought down to 18 months, with a 12-month maximum wait for coronary artery bypass grafts and some associated procedures. The second set of NHS performance tables[6] was published in July, and included details of outpatient waiting times in a range of specialties.

In August, a version of a booklet on *The patient's charter* in relation to services for children and young people was distributed for consultation, with the intention of issuing a final version during 1996. Work is also under way on a similar booklet in relation to mental health services, which should be distributed for consultation in Spring 1996.

The Government's response[7] to the Wilson Committee's report on its review of the NHS complaints procedure[8] was published in March (see page 216). The overall aim of the new complaints procedure will be to resolve complaints quickly and simply, and to ensure that information from them is used to improve services. The intention is to introduce the new procedures from 1 April 1996.

In a primary care-led NHS, decisions about health care are taken as close to patients as possible, with a greater voice for patients and their carers in such decisions. To achieve this, general practitioners (GPs) and their teams are being given a wider scope of influence in the purchasing and provision of health care, within agreed public health priorities. The development of a primary care-led NHS continued during 1995. Primary care involvement in purchasing was strengthened - in particular through expansion of the scope of GP fundholding, introduction of a community fundholding option and pilot studies of total purchasing schemes. The role of health authorities has also been developed, and from 1 April 1996 the new unified authorities will be well placed to develop comprehensive strategies across primary and secondary care. In October, the Secretary of State for Health announced a wide-ranging 'listening exercise' on the future shape of primary care services to identify the range, shape and characteristics of services that patients could receive in the future, and the key obstacles to delivering those services. The results of this consultation will be drawn together in Spring 1996.

(iii)   *Priority setting*

In March, in its response to the Health Select Committee on Priority Setting[9], the Government set out its approach to priority setting at three levels:

— Ministers, advised by the Department of Health (DH), set out a framework of national priorities and targets for improvement through annual priorities and planning guidance to the NHS and through important policies such as the Health of the Nation White Paper[1] and *The patient's charter*[5];

— health authorities and GP fundholders assess the needs of the people they serve and decide what treatments and services are required to meet those needs, informed by proper consultation with the public; *and*

— individual clinicians decide the most clinically appropriate treatment and clinical priority for each patient, based on their assessment of that patient's needs.

NHS treatment is available to everyone on the basis of clinical need, regardless of ability to pay. There should be no clinically effective treatment which a health authority decides as a matter of principle not to provide.

The purpose of the annual priorities and planning guidance is to provide an overall context for the planning and delivery of health services, and to focus the NHS on the most important national priorities - both in the medium term and for the next planning year. The guidance for 1996/97[10], issued on 9 June, was considerably revised to reflect the strategic framework and to give a clearer focus for local NHS planning and priority setting.

The guidance sets out the continuing baseline requirements for the NHS as progress towards the Health of the Nation targets[1], *Patient's charter* standards and guarantees[5], waiting time targets and guarantees, national and local efficiency targets, agreed financial and activity targets and control of drugs expenditure. In addition to these specific output requirements, some important aspects of the infrastructure that supports the NHS require continuous development - in particular, sustained improvement in communications and continued progress in the implementation of the information management and technology strategy. It also details a limited range of medium-term priorities for the NHS - crucial areas which need managerial attention over the next three to five years, including the move towards a primary care-led NHS; mental health services; cost-effectiveness and evidence-based decision-making; involvement of the public, users of NHS services and carers; continuing care services; and human resources. Objectives have been identified for each medium-term priority, framed in a general way to allow local interpretation to suit individual local circumstances. They will be reviewed on an annual basis.

The six main priorities for 1996/97, which are all of equal importance, are:

— to work towards the development of a primary care-led NHS, in which decisions about the purchasing and provision of health care are taken as close to patients as possible;

— in partnership with local authorities, to purchase and monitor a comprehensive range of secure, residential, inpatient and community services to enable people with mental illness to receive effective care and treatment in the most appropriate setting in accordance with their needs;

— to improve the cost effectiveness of services throughout the NHS and thereby secure the greatest health gain from the resources available, through formulating decisions on the basis of appropriate evidence about clinical effectiveness;

— to give greater voice and influence to users of NHS services and their carers in their own care, the development and definition of standards set for NHS services locally and the development of NHS policy both locally and nationally;

— to ensure, in collaboration with local authorities and other organisations, that integrated services are in place to meet needs for continuing health care and to allow elderly, disabled or vulnerable people to be supported in the community; *and*

— to develop NHS organisations as good employers with particular reference to workforce planning, education and training, employment policy and practice, the development of teamwork, reward systems, staff utilisation, and staff welfare.

(iv) *Research and development*

The research and development strategy

Research and development (R&D) is a core function of the NHS and an integral part of the Department's responsibilities. The R&D strategy comprises two complementary programmes: the Department's policy research programme and the NHS R&D programme. The strategy also promotes strong links with the scientific community and with research councils, charities and industry. A national forum has been established to improve liaison and co-operation with other major sources of research funds, including charities and industry.

Policy-related research

The policy research programme provides a knowledge base for strategic matters of health service provision, social services policies and central activity to improve the health of the whole population. The programme supports research across the whole range of Departmental responsibilities. Such research provides evidence-based findings which can advance Health of the Nation objectives[1].

The coronary heart disease (CHD) and stroke key area is supported by research on nutrition, smoking, hypertension and heavy drinking. For mental illness, there are several studies on suicide and on work to identify cost-effective services for mentally ill people. Studies on breast cancer and cervical screening, on the early detection of melanoma, and on smoking in pregnancy and among adolescents support targets for reducing the incidence of cancer. DH is planning to take forward research on variations in health in line with Health of the Nation commitments.

The strategic focus extends to other areas where large research programmes are being developed - including primary health care, air pollution, child care, community health services, prescribing, purchasing, human resources and effectiveness, and vaccine development. Priority setting draws on advice from the Departmental Research Committee chaired by the Director of Research and Development. Membership is drawn from senior policy and professional colleagues, including the Chief Medical Officer.

Developments in the NHS R&D programme

The NHS R&D strategy has a key role to play in the move to strengthen the scientific basis of health care. It encourages NHS managers and health professionals to convert information needs into answerable research questions, and to track down the best evidence to address the problems faced in day-to-day practice. The NHS R&D programme is therefore a priority-led programme driven by the needs of the service.

Over 300 studies have been funded in research programmes on mental health; cancer; cardiovascular disease and stroke; the interface between primary and secondary care; mother and child health; physical and complex disabilities; health technology assessment and ways to implement R&D findings; and consumer input into NHS research programmes. Each programme is expected to last five years (except the health technology assessment programme, which is continuous) and each has a budget of around £5 million. Health technology assessment forms the largest single body of research within the NHS R&D programme, and generates considerable interest in this country and internationally; this initiative includes the evaluation of new technologies, as well as rigorous assessment of existing ones.

Research, however, is not an end in itself; the findings must be made available to everyone who needs to know about them. The R&D information systems strategy has been set up to look at ways to bring information about R&D findings to the attention of clinicians and decision-makers. The Cochrane Database of Systematic Reviews and a new publication, *Effectiveness matters*[11], from the NHS Centre for Reviews and Dissemination at York, are important additions to existing routes for the dissemination of new findings.

Developments in R&D funding

The introduction of the NHS reforms and other organisational changes raised concerns that there might be inadequacies in the NHS's systems for funding and supporting R&D. In response to these concerns, the Government set up a Task Force to examine the funding and support of R&D in the NHS, chaired by Professor Anthony Culyer, Professor of Economics at the University of York.

The Task Force's report was published in September 1994[12], and was widely welcomed. It contained a broad range of recommendations which aimed to improve mechanisms to determine R&D priorities in the NHS; to introduce a single funding source for R&D in all NHS settings; and to provide better management and accountability for NHS resources devoted to R&D. The Government accepted the main recommendations, and an Implementation Plan was published in April 1995[13]. The work on implementation is proceeding according to this plan. R&D activities funded directly by the NHS, and the costs of supporting other research funders' R&D in the NHS, will be funded from 1996/97 by an initial levy on the allocations of health authorities. Trusts have been asked to declare their R&D activity and its costs to the NHS, so that a full levy can be constructed for 1997/98 and subsequent years.

The Central Research and Development Committee has established an implementation group to oversee the development of these new arrangements, and the NHS Executive has established a working party to advise it on the interface between the new R&D funding arrangements and NHS patient care.

House of Lords report on medical research and the NHS reforms

The House of Lords report on medical research and the NHS reforms[14], published in June, endorsed the achievements of the NHS R&D strategy, and said that "of all the NHS reforms since 1990, the R&D strategy is certainly the one least widely known; but among those who are aware of it, it is we suspect, the one most unequivocally welcomed".

The Government response to this report[15], published in September, welcomed the constructive spirit of the report, and reaffirmed the Government's determination to provide the NHS with an environment in which high-quality R&D could flourish; this was reiterated in a subsequent debate in the House of Lords in December.

References

1. Department of Health. *The Health of the Nation: a strategy for health in England.* London: HMSO, 1992 (Cm. 1986).
2. Department of Health. *Caring for people: community care the next decade and beyond.* London: HMSO, 1989 (Cm. 849).
3. Department of Health. *NHS responsibilities for meeting continuing health care needs.* Wetherby (West Yorkshire): Department of Health, 1995 (Health Service Guidelines: HSG(95)8, Local Authority Circular: LAC(95)5).
4. Department of Health. *An introduction to joint commissioning: practical guidance on joint commissioning for project leaders.* Wetherby (West Yorkshire): Department of Health, 1995.
5. Department of Health. *The patient's charter.* London: Department of Health, 1991.
6. Department of Health. *The patient's charter: the NHS performance guide: 1994-95.* Wetherby (West Yorkshire): Department of Health, 1995.

7. Department of Health. *Acting on complaints: the Government's proposals in response to 'Being Heard': the report of the Review Committee on NHS Complaints Procedures.* London: Department of Health, 1995.

8. NHS Executive. *Being heard: the report of a review committee on the NHS complaints procedures.* London: Department of Health, 1995. Chair: Professor Alan Wilson.

9. Department of Health. *Government Response to the First Report from the Health Committee: priority setting in the NHS: purchasing: 1994-95 Session.* London: HMSO, 1995 (Cm. 2826).

10. Department of Health. *Priorities and planning guidance for the NHS: 1996/97.* Wetherby (West Yorkshire): Department of Health, 1995 (Executive Letter: EL(95)68).

11. NHS Centre for Reviews and Dissemination. *Effectiveness matters (vol. 1).* York: University of York, NHS Centre for Reviews and Dissemination, 1995.

12. Research and Development Task Force. *Supporting research and development in the NHS.* London: HMSO, 1994. Chair: Professor Anthony Culyer.

13. Department of Health. *Supporting research and development in the NHS: implementation plan.* Wetherby (West Yorkshire): Department of Health, 1995 (Executive Letter: EL(95)46).

14. House of Lords Select Committee on Science and Technology. *Medical research and the NHS reforms report: 1994-95 Session.* London: HMSO, 1995 (HL Paper 12).

15. Department of Health. *Government Response to the Third Report of the House of Lords Select Committee on Science and Technology: medical research and the NHS reforms: 1994-95 Session.* London: HMSO, 1995 (Cm. 2984).

(b)   Role of the NHS in maintaining public health

(i)   *Public health and the NHS*

The changing role of public health

Public Health in England[1], published in July 1994, outlined the public health functions of health authorities, which would mainly be performed through multidisciplinary departments led by directors of public health (DsPH). The central role of the DPH in the new health authorities has been emphasised by making the postholder one of the three statutory executive members of each authority's management board.

All health authorities are required to make arrangements to involve professionals in the full range of their work. DsPH are pivotal in ensuring that health care professionals contribute to authority decisions, and have a key role themselves in providing public health advice.

Public health specialists are also working closely with primary care colleagues in the development of the primary care-led NHS, including the provision of evidence-based advice for purchasing decisions. In June, a working group on public health in primary care was set up to explore further ways in which public health and primary care professionals can work together for the benefit of patients.

Medical manpower

Changes to health authorities and other developments created a need to look more closely at the likely future demand for public health specialists and the ways in which training needs would be met. A working party with representatives from the Faculty of Public Health Medicine and the British

Medical Association (BMA) was set up to consider these matters, and there were moves to incorporate the specialty of public health medicine into the Standing Workforce Advisory Group process.

Multidisciplinary public health

The development of health authority and GP purchasing has highlighted the need to strengthen multidisciplinary public health practice. The NHS Executive has commissioned the King's Fund Development Centre to review and publish evidence of good practice in this area. Their findings should complement *Making it happen*[2] the recent report of the Standing Nursing and Midwifery Advisory Committee on the public health contribution of nurses, midwives and health visitors (see below).

(ii)   'Making it happen'

Making it happen[2] sets the contribution of nurses, midwives and health visitors within the broader context of achieving the multidisciplinary health objectives of the NHS. Nurses and midwives are key contributors to the provision of health care to individuals. The report reaffirms this role but goes further, noting that they are also a major force in health promotion in local communities.

The knowledge that nurses and midwives have about the personal health of individuals can help to identify more precisely issues of community health need, as well as access and attitude to services. The key recommendations for education and research, communication and information provide an agenda into the future on the ways in which health services can most effectively utilise the role and expertise of nurses and midwives for promoting good health in the community. 'Making it happen' is a joint policy initiative between DH and the Welsh Office; it has been brought to the attention of a number of national bodies and public health and professional organisations. From consultation on the report's recommendations, many note that more progress needs to be made in education, and how NHS employers harness the contribution of nursing professionals in health care and commissioning. Primary responsibility for implementation of the report's recommendations in England lies with health authorities and NHS Trusts, with the support of the Regional Offices of the NHS Executive.

(iii)   Health needs assessment

As in previous years, the assessment of health needs continued to develop as a core activity of District Health Authorities (DHAs). The second series of epidemiologically based health needs assessments, described in last year's Report[3], is nearing completion and publication is anticipated in mid-1996. During 1995, NHS users were asked for their opinions about the first series. Those consulted indicated that it was considered to be very valuable and soundly based, but that more effort should be made to make key points available to a wider audience; comments were also made about a need to update the first series.

As a result of these discussions, prototype summaries are being developed and the Department is seeking further expert advice about the need to update chapters in the first series. Discussions have also taken place about the choice of topics which would most merit attention in a planned third series, which will take account, where appropriate, of changes related to a primary care-led NHS.

Information in the first series of health needs assessments has been mainly used by DHA public health departments for reviews of services, strategic planning and contract specification. These discussions have offered opportunities to involve clinicians in the process of setting contracts, and health needs assessment also forms an important part of a wider strategy to promote clinical effectiveness within the NHS.

(iv)   *National confidential enquiries*

Support for the national confidential enquiries has been steadily increasing over a number of years, reflecting a growing commitment to audit and the importance of accurate data on professional practice. Two reports were published during the year. The National Confidential Enquiry into Peri-operative Deaths (NCEPOD)[4], which covered the year 1992/93, and the Confidential Enquiry into Stillbirths and Deaths in Infancy (CESDI)[5], which covered the calendar year 1993.

NCEPOD made recommendations on critical care services; the supervision of trainees; surgical and anaesthetic experience and skills; laparoscopic procedures; patient transfers; standards of practice; and the quality of medical notes. The CESDI report included recommendations on stillbirths, neonatal and infant mortality, including guidance and training of professionals involved in the care of unborn and newly born babies; resuscitation of the newborn; preparation of necropsy reports; and counselling of bereaved parents.

During the year, work also continued on the enquiries into Maternal Deaths, Homicides and Suicides by Mentally Ill People and Counselling for Genetic Disorders.

(v)   *National Casemix Office and NHS Centre for Coding and Classification*

National Casemix Office

The National Casemix Office has been set up to develop, maintain, issue and market patient grouping tools and classification methodologies for use in the NHS. Such groupings allow patient-based data to be aggregated in various ways to assist in analysis. One type of grouping is by health care resource groups (HRGs) for use in costing, the contracting process and for internal resource management. Other types of groupings, for example health benefit groups (HBGs), enable analysis of epidemiological data to assist purchasers to define needs. The Office has close working relations with the NHS Centre for Coding and Classification, with which it shares a supervisory board responsible for strategic guidance.

The current programme includes:

— refinement of HRGs for inpatients and day cases;

— pilot projects of HRGs in mental health services and the care of elderly people;

— development of HRGs in outpatient and community services;

— pilot projects and continued development of HBGs to inform purchasing;

— support of the extension of HRG costing for district and GP fundholder purchasing in the provision of acute health care;

— provision of casemix-adjusted health service indicators and national HRG statistics; *and*

— support of the implementation of casemix methods in the NHS through training courses, seminars, conferences and help-desk services.

NHS Centre for Coding and Classification

The NHS Centre for Coding and Classification (NHSCCC) continues to maintain and develop the Read Codes - a computerised thesaurus of health care terms and one of the key projects of the information management and technology (IM&T) strategy for the NHS in England (see page 217). The NHSCCC also has responsibility for health care classification and improving the quality of coded clinical data by facilitation of data definitions, standards and training. The NHSCCC has helped to develop a sophisticated computer simulation which can be used to illustrate how information technology can provide access to decision-support systems, and allow clinical information to be shared between health care professionals via an NHS-wide electronic network within the foreseeable future.

The current programme includes:

— work to help to implement the new Read Codes version 3, with the establishment of pilot sites in primary care to explore issues related to the exchange of clinical records using Read Codes;

— development of a range of mapping tables and specific guidance to enable exchange of clinical messages and migration to systems that use Read Codes version 3;

— development of prototype software to show possible approaches for retrieval and analysis of clinical information from systems that use Read Codes version 3;

— improvement of the quality of coded clinical data via implementation of agreed national definitions of primary diagnosis; *and*

— facilitation of the implementation of Read Codes throughout the NHS by the identification of barriers to their use and providing information to users and decision-makers.

(vi)   *Quality of service and effectiveness of care*

The delivery of effective health care services must reflect an up-to-date knowledge and understanding of current research. The making of informed choices likely to deliver the best outcomes is a key component of quality and effectiveness of care for individual patients and their clinicians, and has become a central issue for those concerned with the planning and provision of NHS services.

During 1995, work continued on the development of a framework for improving clinical effectiveness, overseen by the Clinical Outcomes Group (COG). Jointly chaired by the Chief Medical and Nursing Officers, the members of COG include representatives from the professions, managers, researchers and patient interest groups. Sustained improvements in clinical effectiveness depend upon changes in the behaviour of patients, clinicians and managers across the NHS, and work has concentrated on ensuring that:

— there is sufficient information on effectiveness and that it is made available in a way that is accessible and suitable to clinicians, managers and patients;

— there are programmes of local and national action to help to ensure that this information becomes part of routine practice so that it can help to change clinical and managerial behaviour; *and*

— the NHS is able to monitor and demonstrate real improvements in the quality, effectiveness and cost-effectiveness of health care.

All NHS purchasers are required to demonstrate improvements in the effectiveness of services, in particular within the key areas of the Health of the Nation strategy[6]. *Improving the effectiveness of clinical services*, published in December[7], gave health authorities information about clinical guidelines, Effective Health Care Bulletins and the health technology assessment programme. A booklet *Promoting clinical effectiveness* has been developed to support the work of all those involved in identification and review of the effectiveness of clinical services in the NHS, and will be published in early 1996.

Clinical audit has become an increasingly accepted prerequisite of high-quality clinical practice - a major achievement which has been acknowledged by the National Audit Office[8] and the Public Accounts Committee. After a tendering exercise, the contract to run a national information and dissemination centre for clinical audit was awarded to a partnership led by the BMA and the Royal

College of Nursing. The new centre will help to spread and promote examples of best practice gained from local initiatives and experiences in audit.

Work is in hand to evaluate the processes and outcomes of medical and clinical audit programmes and new management arrangements have been put into place to reflect the changing nature of management in the NHS. *The new health authorities and the clinical audit initiative*[9], issued in October, described how clinical audit can be developed in a primary care-led NHS, the monitoring roles of the Regional Offices and the responsibilities of health authority management.

(vii)   Clinical and health outcomes

Health outcome indicators

A revised and updated version of the first set of Population Health Outcome Indicators[10,11] was published as part of the public health common data set (PHCDS) in December[12], and also included additional indicators for hip replacement surgery and mental health. The Wessex Institute of Public Health was commissioned by the Central Health Outcomes Unit (CHOU) to survey the use of health outcomes assessment and of these indicators by health authorities. A telephone survey was carried out during late 1995; a report is expected during Spring 1996, to be followed by a compilation of case studies from a selection of districts.

Following a workshop in January, ten topics were selected for the development of new outcome indicators: asthma, hypertension/stroke, severe mental illness, one cancer, fractured neck of femur, myocardial infarction, diabetes mellitus, cataract, continence and pregnancy/childbirth. Working groups that included clinicians, managers, policy-makers, patient representatives, researchers and others were set up during the year to start work on these indicators, supported by the UK Clearing House on Health Outcomes, the Clinical Accountability Service Planning and Evaluation group (CASPE), the Centre for Reviews and Dissemination and the Royal College of Physicians of London, and co-ordinated by Anglia and Oxford Region. Substantial progress was made on the pilot topic, asthma, and a report is due early in 1996. The rest of the working groups will report by March 1997.

Further work was undertaken to develop a time series of national composite health outcome indicators. Benchmark values for each indicator used in the composite were based on the best value achieved by any district in England during 1992.

Clinical indicators

A first set of 14 clinical indicators, reflecting aspects of clinical care that may raise questions about the quality of care for further investigation, was recommended by a combined Joint Consultants Committee/NHS Executive working group in May. Pilot studies of these indicators will occur during 1996.

A further set of such indicators is under development, drawing on special data sets - for example from the Major Trauma Outcomes Study and cancer registries.

Rationalisation of indicators

In November, the CHOU issued a consultation document to users of the PHCDS which contained proposals to draw together clinical, health and outcomes indicators from a variety of existing data sets into one, structured set. Based on the results of this consultation, the CHOU proposes to: review all existing indicators; remove duplicate or unnecessary indicators; re-specify each indicator by use of a new template; and develop an electronic database and compendium of indicators. Such rationalisation will also provide a baseline for more targeted development of future indicators, to fill in defined gaps in existing data sets.

Outcomes projects

Alongside its own extensive programme to develop outcome indicators, the CHOU supports a number of projects which aim to develop the methods and information systems necessary to create new indicators; several projects were completed during 1995. These included: an investigation into variation in hospitalisation rates for 45 selected medical conditions and 32 surgical procedures; the development of EUROQoL, an instrument to measure general health and well-being; a reliability and validation study of Functional Assessment of Care Environment (FACE), a structured electronic record used to describe physical and mental health, social well-being, the care environment and interventions for people with mental illness and learning disabilities; the development of the Health of the Nation Outcome Scale (HoNOS, a scale for monitoring progress with the mental health key area of the Health of the Nation initiative[6]); and the development of a set of mental health indicators by use of ten-year linked follow-up data from the Oxford Record Linkage study.

(viii)   Regional epidemiological services for communicable disease

Reorganisation of the NHS provided an opportunity to review the provision of regional epidemiological services for communicable disease and to gather together the inevitably different kinds of service provided. *Public health in England*[1], published in July 1994, reaffirmed that surveillance, prevention and control of communicable disease would remain a fundamental public health task, and that Regional Directors of Public Health would continue to be responsible for ensuring that this public health function was discharged effectively in their Region.

A national Service Level Agreement with the Public Health Laboratory Service (PHLS) was signed in November 1995 and will come into effect on 1 April 1996. The key objectives of the new service are to enable regions and health authorities to discharge their responsibilities in relation to communicable diseases and to tailor the service to meet local needs, whilst also providing via the PHLS a consistent and coherent approach to communicable disease across England (see page 211).

References

1. Department of Health. *Public health in England: roles and responsibilities of the Department of Health and the NHS.* London: Department of Health, 1994.
2. Department of Health. *Making it happen: the contribution, role and development of nurses, midwives and health visitors: report of the Standing Nursing and Midwifery Advisory Committee.* Wetherby (West Yorkshire): Department of Health, 1995 (Executive Letter: EL(95)58).
3. Department of Health. *On the State of the Public Health: the annual report of the Chief Medical Officer of the Department of Health for the year* 1994. London: HMSO, 1995; 128.
4. National Confidential Enquiry into Peri-operative Deaths. *The Report of the National Confidential Enquiry into Peri-operative Deaths.* London: National Confidential Enquiry into Peri-operative Deaths, 1994.
5. National Advisory Body on the Confidential Enquiry. *Report of the Confidential Enquiry into Stillbirths and Deaths in Infancy (CESDI): 1 January-1 December.* London: Department of Health, 1995.
6. Department of Health. *The Health of the Nation: a strategy for health in England.* London: HMSO, 1992 (Cm. 1986).
7. Department of Health. *Improving the effectiveness of clinical services.* Wetherby (West Yorkshire): Department of Health, 1995 (Executive Letter: EL(95)105).
8. National Audit Office. *Clinical audit in England: report by the Comptroller and Auditor General.* London: HMSO, 1995.
9. Department of Health. *The new health authorities and the clinical audit initiative: outline of planned monitoring arrangements.* Wetherby (West Yorkshire): Department of Health, 1995 (Executive Letter: EL(95)103).
10. Department of Health. *Population health outcome indicators for the NHS: 1993: England: a consultation document.* London: Department of Health, 1993.
11. Department of Health. *On the State of the Public Health: the annual report of the Chief Medical Officer of the Department of Health for the year 1994.* London: HMSO, 1995; 132.
12. Department of Health. *Public health common data set 1995: incorporating health outcome indicators from the NHS: data definitions and user guide: vol 2.* Guildford: University of Surrey, Institute of Public Health, 1995.

(c)   Primary health care

(i)   Organisation of primary care

Clinical practice continues to change to meet demand. Organisationally, the policy of an NHS led by primary care - with provision of more services closer to patients, increased influence of GPs on providers of secondary care, and alliances for care with other caring services - is in the vanguard of such change.

GP fundholding continues to help to bring about change in working practices in secondary care, with health gain for patients. Total purchasing schemes have led to improved services in some localities and multifunds (groups of autonomous fundholding practices who work together with common objectives) and commissioning have supported improved services and encouraged GPs to work closely together to bring change.

The Department has worked with the profession to reduce bureaucracy in general practice. *Patients not paper*[1], the report of the efficiency scrutiny into bureaucracy in general practice, was published in June. Its main recommendations were: to rationalise claim forms and payment procedures (this will result in a reduction of 17 million forms annually in England and Wales); to make best use of information technology; and to help practices to help themselves.

Professionals have led the development of innovative models in out-of-hours care. There are now improved working practices for the profession and the extension of collaborative working - such as a new primary care emergency centre based at Southport District General Hospital.

(ii)   Prescribing

NHS expenditure on drugs, dressings and appliances prescribed by GPs increased by 9.5% in 1994/95 - a smaller increase than in recent years, but still faster than other areas of NHS spending. Changes in 1995 included generic prescribing reaching 56% of all prescriptions issued, a 13% increase in usage of inhaled steroids for asthma prophylaxis, and further falls in the prescribing of benzodiazepines and drugs of limited clinical value. Major increases in prescribing and cost were seen for proton-pump-inhibitor anti-ulcer drugs and selective serotonin-reuptake inhibitor (SSRI) antidepressants; as with all drugs, these should be used thoughtfully where their properties add real value.

GP fundholders continue to make cost improvements and the incentive scheme for non-fundholders has led to more effective prescribing with estimated savings of £30 million annually. A revised method to allocate prescribing budgets to health authorities - including a needs-based weighting factor - was developed in consultation with the medical profession and others. Health authorities discussed with GP representatives how to apply flexibility in setting practice budgets.

PRODIGY is a computerised point-of-consultation system to support therapeutic decision-making. One hundred and fifty practices are taking part in a research and development project to evaluate its effects on GPs' prescribing and to obtain the views of doctors and patients alike. If successful, the project could help towards development of a comprehensive point-of-consultation decision-support system. Other important developments in information technology included the launch of the first electronic version of the *British National Formulary*, and electronic access to drug data for health authorities (see page 217).

Following wide consultation, guidance on the managed introduction of a new drug - interferon beta lb for multiple sclerosis - was issued in association with clinical guidance from the Standing Medical Advisory Committee (SMAC)[2] to achieve clinically appropriate targeting of the treatment and follow-up of long-term effects.

Results from the eight nurse prescribing demonstration practices confirmed the practicability of this initiative. A wider evaluation involving all practices in a health authority will start in April 1996, in Bolton.

A review of the needs of prescribers, health authorities and the NHS for centrally provided prescribing information, education and training was commissioned by the Department. The report commended the Medicines Resource Centre (MeReC), the Medical Advisors Support Centre, the Prescribing Research Unit and the Management Services Information Systems Development Unit for their previous work. However, the changing organisation and culture of general practice and health authorities indicated a need for a more integrated approach with a wider remit. Ministers agreed to implement the report's recommendations by replacing these units with two new bodies, the National Prescribing Development Centre and the Prescribing Support Unit.

(iii)   Professional development and clinical audit

The Clinical Outcomes Group (COG) published the report of the primary health care clinical audit working group in January[3]. This set a strategic direction for clinical audit and quality assurance in primary care. It considered audit among all primary health care professionals, and included sections on multiprofessional audit, the use of clinical guidelines, links with research and development and continuing education, commissioning for audit, user focus, and audit and service development.

Studies provided examples of audits leading to improved quality of care and outcomes for patients. Audit groups made a considerable contribution to improving clinical effectiveness by encouraging the use of evidence-based audit protocols. Audit groups comprise many experienced and skilled staff who train and support primary health care teams to carry out audit and help with important aspects of audit such as multiprofessional team working, management of change, information technology, critical appraisal and guidelines, and significant event audit. Although audit continues to be led by primary care clinicians, primary care audit groups are now working closely with health authorities on joint objectives.

Some audit groups have improved their links with programmes for continuing education, professional development and research. For example, South Tyneside medical audit advisory group organised a district-wide audit and education programme on the use of aspirin by GPs and hospitals for patients with acute myocardial infarction, accompanied by a publicity campaign for patients to encourage the long-term use of aspirin after myocardial infarction. Some regional advisers are encouraging practice and personal education plans. A training package is available for clinical tutors and clinical audit staff to assist practices to formulate plans for continuing professional development.

References

1. NHS Executive. *Patients not paper: report of the efficiency scrutiny into bureaucracy in general practice.* Wetherby (West Yorkshire): Department of Health, 1995.
2. Department of Health. Interferon beta. *CMO's Update* 1995; **9:** 3.
3. NHS Executive. *Clinical audit in primary health care.* Wetherby (West Yorkshire): Department of Health, 1995.

(d)   Specialised clinical services

(i)   *Specialised services*

Following consultation on the Chief Medical Officer's internal review of the purchasing of specialised services, the establishment of the National Specialist Commissioning Advisory Group (NSCAG) was recommended, with the following terms of reference:

— to run the Supra-Regional services arrangements as now;

— to identify the small number of other highly specialised services that require central purchasing;

— to identify service developments in the evaluation stage, for which it may pay the service costs; *and*

— to secure the production of purchasing guidelines to assist local purchasers.

In May, Ministers agreed to the NSCAG's terms of reference and membership; the Group held its first meeting in November and will take over from the Supra-Regional Services Advisory Group on 1 April 1996.

(ii)   *Cancer*

The overall incidence of cancer is rising, consistent with an ageing population; this observation, together with variations in cancer services provision across the country, led to the setting up of an Expert Advisory Group on Cancer to advise on the organisation of cancer services[1]. On 24 April, after wide consultation, the then Secretary of State for Health unveiled a strategic framework for the future development of cancer services based on the Group's report *A policy framework for commissioning cancer services*[2].

This report recommends that cancer services should be organised at three levels, with primary care seen as the focus of care; cancer units created in many local hospitals of a sufficient size to support a multidisciplinary team with the expertise and facilities to treat commoner cancers; and cancer centres situated in larger hospitals to treat less common cancers and to support smaller cancer units by providing services (including radiotherapy) that are not available in all local hospitals. Key principles emphasise a patient-centred approach to ensure that all patients have access to high-quality care wherever they live, to ensure optimum cure rates and quality of life. Further guidance on implementation will be issued early in 1996 to include timescales, relative roles and responsibilities, and aspects of specialisation.

(iii)   *Minimal access therapy*

Thanks to a generous donation from the Wolfson Foundation, matched by money from central funds, two facilities for training in minimal access therapy were formally opened. Mr Gerald Malone MP, the Minister for Health, opened the Minimal Access Therapy Training Unit (MATTU) at the Royal College of Surgeons of England, and the Hon Tom Sackville MP, then Parliamentary Under Secretary of State for Health in the House of Commons, attended the opening of the Leeds Institute for Minimally Invasive Therapy (LIMIT). These two centres are now well established, and provide a range of courses at basic, intermediate and advanced levels.

During the year, the profession agreed that standards for courses run by the centres and those organised elsewhere in NHS hospitals should be judged against a single yardstick. As a result, the MATTU, the LIMIT and the Minimal Access Therapy Training Unit in Scotland, in consultation with the Association of Endoscopic Surgeons of Great Britain and Ireland, now specify the content of courses. Those that are suitable are recognised by the appropriate Royal College.

(iv)   Osteoporosis

The Department published the report of the Advisory Group on Osteoporosis[3] on 31 January; its terms of reference were: "To establish what information about osteoporosis is available, what research is being conducted and what further work needs to be done, and to report to Ministers".

The Advisory Group was chaired by Professor David Barlow and included clinicians, and representatives of the Royal Colleges of Nursing and of General Practitioners and of the National Osteoporosis Society, representing patients. The key recommendations of the report are that:

— although population screening for osteoporosis is not appropriate, nevertheless bone scans should be available for women already identified to be at high risk of developing osteoporosis;

— national clinical guidelines for the treatment of osteoporosis should be developed;

— specific further research should be carried out;

— professional and public education is needed; and

— improved co-ordination and communication between specialists should be encouraged.

The report was endorsed by Ministers and the SMAC, and was circulated to all NHS bodies. The Royal College of Physicians of London will co-ordinate the development of national clinical guidelines for osteoporosis, as recommended in the report. The Department also increased its financial support for the National Osteoporosis Society, in recognition of its important role in patient and professional education.

(v)   Transplantation

Although about 2,700 organ transplants now take place every year, the number of patients waiting for such interventions continues to rise. The shortage of donor organs reflects increasing demand, as more patients are identified who might benefit from a transplant, and also the fall in the main source of supply with the continued reduction in fatal road accidents. About one-quarter of potential donors are lost because relatives feel unable to consent to organ removal. Research indicates that where a prior intention to donate organs in the event of death is known to relatives, few will refuse consent. In 1994, Ministers therefore decided to establish a permanent computerised register which would hold a confidential record of people who wish to donate their organs, and which would be available for local transplant co-ordinators to check at any time. By December 1995, 2.25 million people had registered.

During the year, it became apparent that developments in the field of xenotransplantation indicated that clinical trials in human beings could take place during 1996. The Secretary of State for Health established an Advisory Group on the Ethics of Xenotransplantation, chaired by Professor Ian Kennedy, Professor of Medical Law and Ethics at King's College, London, to provide advice on the ethical issues raised by xenotransplantation procedures. The Advisory Group's terms of reference are: "In the light of recent and potential developments in xenotransplantation, to review the acceptability of and ethical framework within which xenotransplantation may be undertaken and to make recommendations". Members of the Group include experts across a wide range of disciplines relevant to xenotransplantation. They started work in December and will report to the Secretary of State for Health during Summer, 1996.

(vi)   Strategic Review of Pathology Services

The report of the Strategic Review of Pathology Services was published in September[4]. This review took two years and looked at current provision of pathology services against the background of the introduction of the NHS internal market, the market testing mechanism, provision of pathology services by the independent sector and technological changes. There was a feeling, prompted in part by Audit Commission reports[5,6], that the cost-effectiveness of pathology services could perhaps be improved. The recommendations of the review were intended to safeguard or improve pathology services without being prescriptive. The review described a number of different organisational changes which might be feasible and effective; while it did not advocate particular arrangements, the review was clear that a pathology service should be professionally directed by a consultant pathologist or clinical scientist of equivalent standing. Market testing was an important tool - but in the case of clinical services, including pathology, the market included other NHS units as well as independent contractors. While a private sector contribution to the provision of clinical services is possible, it should only go ahead if strong clinical support exists. Ministers welcomed the report and commended it to all who are concerned with NHS pathology services.

(vii)   Intensive care

A professional and Departmental Working Group set up to recommend guidelines on admission to and discharge from intensive-care and high-dependency-care units completed its work at the end of 1995. Guidelines intended to help hospital clinicians to decide which patients should be referred for intensive care will be issued in Spring, 1996. The guidelines will point to the important role played by high-dependency care as an intermediate level between general wards and intensive care. Important factors in considering admission include the source of referral, the reversibility of the patient's illness, the patient's pre-existing health and the need for advanced respiratory support. In order to make the most effective use of these costly facilities, patients should be discharged as soon as their condition has been treated and improved. Since intensive-care units inevitably experience considerable fluctuations in demand, transfers between units are likely to be needed during periods of peak demand, and guidance on how to ensure that necessary transfers can be achieved safely will be included.

(viii)   *Emergency admissions*

There was further evidence of a rising trend in the number of emergency admissions to hospitals. In general and acute hospital beds in England there was a rise of 300,000 over five years, from 2.95 million in 1990/91 to 3.25 million in 1994/95 (see Figure 5.1). There are considerable, often very localised, variations and no single or major cause has been identified. The largest numerical rise was in patients admitted in the diagnostic group covering general symptoms and ill-defined conditions. There was an increase of 250,000 patients who stayed in hospital for 48 hours or less.

Figure 5.1: *General and acute emergency admissions: average daily number by month, England, 1990/91-1994/95*

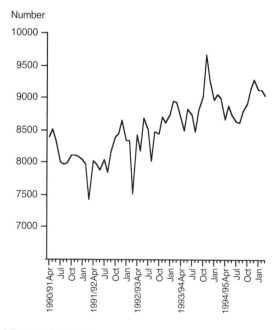

Source: Hospital Episode Statistics

146

The pattern of an increasing rate of emergency admissions coupled with the changing nature of elective inpatient treatment, as more patients are treated on a day-case basis, will need to be planned for and managed.

References

1. Department of Health. *On the State of the Public Health: the annual report of the Chief Medical Officer of the Department of Health for the year 1994.* London: HMSO, 1995; 137.
2. Department of Health, Welsh Office. *A policy framework for commissioning cancer services: a report by the Expert Advisory Group on Cancer to the Chief Medical Officers of England and Wales: guidance for purchasers and providers of cancer services.* London: Department of Health, 1995.
3. Department of Health. *Advisory Group on Osteoporosis: report.* London: Department of Health, 1994. Chair: Professor David Barlow.
4. Department of Health. *Strategic review of pathology services.* London: HMSO, 1995.
5. Audit Commission. *The pathology services: a management review.* London: HMSO, 1991.
6. Audit Commission. *Critical path: an analysis of the pathology services.* London: HMSO, 1993.

(e)   Maternity and child health services

(i)   Implementation of 'Changing Childbirth'

Since the Government's acceptance, in January 1994, of the Expert Maternity Group's report, *Changing childbirth*[1], the NHS has worked to implement the report's recommendations over a five-year timescale[2,3]. During 1995, the Changing Childbirth Implementation Team visited providers of maternity care and purchasers of such care throughout the country, and found that good progress was being made. An Advisory Group met to consider issues about implementation, and agreed to hold a conference in 1996 to examine educational and training matters.

During the year, £1 million were allocated to support a further 24 development projects covering a broad range of issues; a video was commissioned for professionals who provide maternity care to show the different ways in which 'Changing Childbirth' is being put into practice; and planning began for a consumer awareness campaign to take place in 1996. DH also supported two multidisciplinary workshops to consider the provision of unbiased information and risk assessment during pregnancy; these workshops were attended by representatives of all the main professional bodies and consumer groups, and much common ground was found. Work began to monitor progress in the NHS against ten key indicators of success; methods of monitoring were developed, and a workshop was held with staff from the 13 sites involved in a pilot scheme.

(ii)   Folic acid and prevention of neural tube defects

In June, DH awarded a contract to the Health Education Authority (HEA) to run a folic acid awareness campaign over the next $2\frac{1}{2}$ years. This will reflect the guidance in the 1992 expert report *Folic acid and the prevention of neural tube defects*[4]. Three means to encourage women to increase their intake of this vitamin will be promoted: by a daily supplement of 400 micrograms of folic acid; by choice of foods which are fortified with folic acid, such as breads and breakfast cereals; and by modifying the diet to include more foods naturally rich in folate. These dietary changes should begin before conception.

Health professionals were the first target group in the campaign and a programme of education was launched in November. It included six seminars at sites throughout England. Guidance for health service purchasers and providers was distributed in preparation for the public launch of the campaign, due to take place on 28 February 1996. A programme of future education will focus on women who may become pregnant, whether planned or non-planned, and on the manufacturers and suppliers of food and dietary supplements.

An Expert Group will be set up by the Committee on Medical Aspects of Food Policy (COMA) to assess and report on the health aspects of increasing folate/folic acid intakes.

(iii)   Sudden infant death syndrome

Last year's Report[5] recorded the continued fall in mortality from sudden infant death syndrome (SIDS) to 1993; the low rate continued in 1994 at 0.6 per 1,000 live births. Meanwhile, case-control studies on sudden deaths in infancy, which are part of the Confidential Enquiry into Stillbirths and Deaths in Infancy (see page 135), are examining the circumstances in which SIDS now occurs and the associated factors. The findings of this work will be reported in Summer, 1996.

In 1994, the Chief Medical Officer set up an Expert Group, chaired by Lady Limerick, to review and re-examine suggestions that the primary cause of SIDS was poisoning by gaseous phosphines, arsines and stibines generated by the action of micro-organisms upon cot mattresses[6]. Following studies carried out by the Public Health Laboratory in Bristol, and the Trace Element Analysis Unit at Southampton General Hospital, the Group concluded that so far there was no evidence to support the hypothesis that chemicals in polyvinylchloride (PVC) mattresses were converted into toxic gases by the growth of micro-organisms. Findings were announced in an interim statement from the Expert Group, but further data from other studies that have been set in train need to be available and assessed before a final report can be produced. At all stages of their deliberations the Expert Group have asked the question "is there any evidence of risk to infants?"; they report that to date they have seen none.

(iv)   Prophylaxis of vitamin K deficiency bleeding in infants

The Reports for 1993[7] and 1994[8] drew attention to a number of new studies into the reported carcinogenic effects of vitamin K. In July 1994, the Chief Medical Officer met representatives of medical and nursing professional bodies to discuss issues related to the administration of vitamin K. Concerns raised included the propriety of administering vitamin K by mouth when it was unlicensed for this route; the likely delay before a licensed oral vitamin K preparation would be available; variations in clinical policy and practice, and in the provision of guidance and local protocols; the possible increased risk of bleeding in some children given vitamin K orally, compared with intramuscular administration; and concerns about the consistency of practice in giving timely information to parents to enable them to give informed consent.

The meeting agreed that advice setting out good practice could best be prepared by the relevant professions. This advice should set out: the basis for vitamin K prophylaxis; the status of existing research findings and impending studies; the importance of early identification and referral of children at risk of vitamin K deficiency bleeding; and the need for agreed and known local policies and practice, including the content and availability of information for parents. The subject was kept under review during 1995, and research findings are now expected to be published in 1996.

(v)   Retinopathy of prematurity

Last year's Report[9] recorded that a nationwide research, training and audit programme on retinopathy of prematurity would begin in 1995. A report of progress during the first year should be available for next year's Report.

(vi)   Paediatric intensive care

Following publication of *The care of critically ill children*[10], the report of a multidisciplinary working party on paediatric intensive care, the NHS Executive commissioned a review by the NHS Centre for Reviews and Dissemination (CRD) to complement the report[11,12]. This review looked at the weight of evidence available to support the conclusions and recommendations of the report, and drew attention to deficiencies in the information available for the UK in regard to the numbers of critically ill children, measures of illness severity, the content of care, and outcomes; it also pointed to the small amount of relevant health services research that had been published. The report, the review and observations of international groups revealed a diversity of opinion on the required level of provision of services, the optimum size of units and their disposition, and their patterns of staffing, but did help to identify areas where there is a lack of research evidence. The differences of opinion did not extend to the clinical or pastoral needs of very sick children and their families. Research on these issues is being incorporated in the NHS R&D programme to enable a more informed discussion about the factors which influence the survival of critically ill children, such as the development of casemix and outcome measures; the identification of ways to determine the impact of qualitative and organisational aspects of intensive care; ways to ensure increased accuracy of cost estimation; and the implications of developments in paediatric intensive care for postgraduate medical education and for children's nurses and their training.

(vii)   Congenital anomalies

In 1993, the Medical Advisory Committee of the Registrar General of the Office of Population Censuses and Surveys (OPCS, to become part of the Office for

National Statistics [ONS] in 1996) set up a working group to review the operation of the notification system which had been set up to monitor congenital malformations. The working group reported in 1995[13].

Among the recommendations of the working group were that:

— for reasons of safeguarding the public health, there should be a two-tier system of receiving and processing notification of congenital anomalies. The first tier would be similar to the present system of rapid surveillance of malformations detected in live births or stillbirths within 10 days of birth. To this tier should be added a second tier of notifications received after this age limit, thus setting up a more complete national database to be used for the monitoring of small area statistics with a view to the identification of new putative hazards and allowing confirmation of their effects; to monitor the effectiveness of preventive interventions on a national scale; and to help with the planning and evaluation of service provision for affected individuals;

— subject to requirements on confidentiality, data on legal abortions which have been carried out on the grounds that there is a substantial risk that, if the child were born, it would suffer from such physical or mental abnormality as to be seriously handicapped should be added to corresponding data from notifications of congenital anomalies and registration of deaths;

— in the implementation of the proposed new system OPCS/ONS, together with collaborating NHS bodies, should seek solutions which will meet current confidentiality requirements and guidance, and that the need to safeguard confidentiality requires adequate systems for handling and processing data to be in place;

— the possibility of electronic capture of anomaly data from birth notifications should be explored;

— where good congenital malformation registers exist outside OPCS/ONS, information should be exchanged with these to improve the completeness and validity of both local and national data, and that loss of local registers would detract from the overall quantity and quality of data on congenital anomalies;

— the possibility of receiving direct notifications from the laboratories that carry out diagnostic tests for chromosomal anomalies and certain genetically determined metabolic disorders, as well as centres specialising in the care of children born with cardiac, neurological and orthopaedic defects, should be considered;

— the name of the OPCS/ONS system should be changed to 'Congenital anomaly system'; *and*

— future methods of coding and classification to be used for congenital malformations and anomalies, with particular reference to current developments outside OPCS/ONS and the problems of syndromes and multiple malformations, should be explored.

The deliberations of the Working Group have already influenced implementation of the OPCS/ONS information technology strategy, and developments in diagnostic classification, encoding and analysis.

References

1. Department of Health. *Changing childbirth: part 1: report of the Expert Maternity Group.* London: HMSO, 1993. Chair: Baroness Cumberlege.
2. Department of Health. *Women-centred maternity services.* Wetherby (West Yorkshire): Department of Health, 1994 (Executive Letter: EL(94)9).
3. Department of Health. *On the State of the Public Health: the annual report of the Chief Medical Officer of the Department of Health for the year 1994.* London: HMSO, 1995; 146.
4. Department of Health. *Folic acid and the prevention of neural tube defects.* London: Department of Health, 1992.
5. Department of Health. *On the State of the Public Health: the annual report of the Chief Medical Officer of the Department of Health for the year 1994.* London: HMSO, 1995; 148.
6. Department of Health. *Expert Group to investigate cot death theories.* London: Department of Health, 1994 (Press Release: H94/553).
7. Department of Health. *On the State of the Public Health: the annual report of the Chief Medical Officer of the Department of Health for the year 1993.* London: HMSO, 1994; 132-3.
8. Department of Health. *On the State of the Public Health: the annual report of the Chief Medical Officer of the Department of Health for the year 1994.* London: HMSO, 1995; 148-9.
9. Department of Health. *On the State of the Public Health: the annual report of the Chief Medical Officer of the Department of Health for the year 1994.* London: HMSO, 1995; 149.
10. Fleming P, Matthew D. *The care of critically ill children: report of the Multidisciplinary Working Party of Paediatric Intensive Care convened by the British Paediatric Association.* London: British Paediatric Association, 1993.
11. NHS Centre for Reviews and Dissemination. *Which way forward for the care of critically ill children?* York: NHS Centre for Reviews and Dissemination, University of York, 1994.
12. Department of Health. *On the State of the Public Health: the annual report of the Chief Medical Officer of the Department of Health for the year 1994.* London: HMSO, 1995; 150.
13. Office of Population Censuses and Surveys. *The OPCS monitoring scheme for congenital malformations: a review by a working group of the Registrar General's Medical Advisory Committee.* London: HMSO, 1995 (Occasional paper no. 43).

(f)   Asthma

A shared concern about the increasing prevalence of asthma prompted DH, in association with the Department of the Environment (DoE), the Institute for Environment and Health (IEH) and the National Asthma Campaign, to organise a one-day conference in November on the possible causes and successful management of asthma. It was addressed by the Hon Tom Sackville MP, then Parliamentary Under Secretary of State for Health in the House of Commons, and Mr James Clappison MP, Parliamentary Under Secretary of State for the Environment in the House of Commons. The invited audience included voluntary organisations, health professionals and the media. Aspects of management addressed included treatment and management in primary care and in the home, in schools and in the workplace.

The conference confirmed that many unanswered questions about the causes of asthma remain. The IEH produced a report, *Understanding asthma*[1], based on the conference session about possible causes and the extent of the problem. In October, DH published the report of the Committee on the Medical Effects of Air Pollutants (COMEAP) on asthma and outdoor air pollution, which concluded that outdoor air pollution does not cause asthma but may aggravate symptoms in a small proportion of patients with asthma (see page 184).

Also in October, DH published the report of a multidisciplinary advisory group which identified ten top research and development priorities for the NHS on asthma management. This research strategy will be taken forward by the NHS research and development programme in collaboration with the National Asthma Campaign.

Reference

1. Institute for Environment and Health. *Understanding asthma.* Leicester: Institute for Environment and Health, 1995.

(g)   Diabetes mellitus

The final report of the joint DH/British Diabetic Association (BDA) St Vincent Task Force for Diabetes was presented to the parent bodies in July[1]. To implement its recommendations within the NHS, the Department set up a diabetes sub-group of the COG; the specific remit of this sub-group is to develop service guidance for purchasers. Initially it has been asked to prepare guidance in three key areas of prevention: diabetic retinopathy and blindness, foot complications and nephropathy.

Membership of the sub-group is composed of senior managers, medical and nursing professionals, representatives of the St Vincent Task Force and the BDA, and several lay members. The sub-group began work in the Autumn and has met at monthly intervals; two processes in pursuing its objectives have been identified. In phase one, it will highlight key features for commissioners of health care, which concentrate on the managerial framework needed to deliver clinically effective care to the population; and, in phase two, it will review guidance currently available and produce new guidance on the priorities for provision of clinically effective care.

Reference

1. Department of Health, British Diabetic Association. *St Vincent Joint Task Force for Diabetes: the report: 1995.* London: Department of Health, 1995.

(h)   Complementary medicine

Work progressed towards the establishment of the General Osteopathic Council, under the Osteopaths Act 1993[1], and the General Chiropractic Council, under the Chiropractors Act 1994[2]. Both these new Councils, which will develop, promote and regulate their respective professions, are expected to be established by mid-1996.

No other complementary therapy group made major progress in 1995 towards similar statutory regulation, but interest in the provision of complementary therapies within the NHS appears to be increasing. A DH-funded report from the

Medical Care Research Unit at the University of Sheffield[3] indicated that some 40% of GP partnerships in England provide access to some form of complementary therapy for their NHS patients. The most frequently provided services were homoeopathy and acupuncture, and GP fundholders were more likely than non-fundholders to offer complementary therapy services to their patients. A follow-up study has been commissioned.

References

1. *Osteopaths Act 1993.* London: HMSO, 1993.
2. *Chiropractors Act 1994.* London: HMSO, 1994.
3. Thomas K, Fall M, Parry G. Nicholl J. *National survey of access to complementary health care via general practice.* Sheffield: Medical Care Research Unit, University of Sheffield, 1995.

(i)   Disability and rehabilitation

During 1995, there were further developments in the areas of disability and rehabilitation. National Continence Day was held in March to increase awareness of and remove some of the taboos that surround the subject and to encourage people to seek help. A further National Continence Day and Bedwetting Day will be held on 19 and 20 March, 1996.

At the beginning of the year, DH officials began work on a programme of co-ordinated initiatives on epilepsy[1]. As part of these initiatives, during National Epilepsy Week in May, the Department held a conference on epilepsy with the theme of 'Youth, users of services and primary care'; work continues on these initiatives.

The NHS *Priorities and planning guidelines* for 1995/96[2] asked local purchasers of health services to improve services for physically disabled people.

A video was produced on pressure sore prevention, aimed at care assistants in residential care and nursing homes. The video, entitled 'Don't get sore - get moving' was also shown on BBC Select (to be known as BBC Focus) on several occasions during the year. In July, the report was issued of a conference entitled 'Pressure sores: using information'[3].

DH continued to fund 12 projects to improve NHS rehabilitation services for people who have suffered brain injury. Research continued into the development of measurable targets for the improvement of services for people with speech and language impairment, pressure sores, hearing disability, and urinary incontinence; into the quality of care of hip fracture patients; and into avoidable amputations in patients with diabetes mellitus.

From 1 April 1995, responsibility for the issue of environmental control systems for severely disabled people was devolved to health authorities. The Advisory Group on Rehabilitation met on four occasions, including its last meeting at the end of 1995; as its final piece of work the Group considered a handbook on rehabilitation, which will be published in 1996.

References

1. Department of Health. *A positive approach to epilepsy.* Wetherby (West Yorkshire): Department of Health, 1995 (Executive Letter: EL(95)120).
2. NHS Executive. *Priorities and planning guidance for the NHS: 1995/96.* Wetherby (West Yorkshire): Department of Health, 1995 (Executive Letter EL(94)55).
3. NHS Executive Information Management Group. *Pressure sores: using information.* Huntingdon: Information Point, Register of Computer Applications, Cambridge and Huntingdon Health Commission, 1995.

(j)   Prison health care

In April, the Prison Service launched its national drugs strategy, *Drug misuse in prison*[1], in line with the Government's White Paper *Tackling drugs together*[2]. Since then, every prison has produced its own local strategy which seeks to achieve a balanced approach to this challenge, focusing on three main areas. Firstly, measures to reduce supply, with improved searching and mandatory drug testing to assist in deterrence from drug misuse and to provide improved information about the incidence of drug misuse in prisons. Secondly, measures to reduce demand and to rehabilitate drug misusers, with a range of pilot treatment programmes introduced in 22 establishments during 1995, including therapeutic communities, detoxification units, and education and counselling services. Thirdly, measures to reduce the potential for damage to the health of prisoners, staff and the wider community that may arise from the misuse of drugs - for example by enhancement of education and counselling services.

The recent increase in the number of mentally disordered prisoners transferred to psychiatric hospitals as restricted patients under sections 47 and 48 of the Mental Health Act 1983[3] was maintained, with 784 transfers in 1995. A sub-committee of the Health Advisory Committee set up to look into the provision of mental health care in prisons held several meetings, and was expected to submit a final report, with recommendations, early in 1996. A Prison Service representative was appointed to serve on the new High Security Psychiatric Services Commissioning Board, which was due to assume on 1 April 1996 the commissioning element of the functions of the Special Hospitals Service Authority. The final report of a study by researchers from the Institute of Psychiatry of the prevalence of mental disorder among the remanded prison population of England and Wales was received, and is expected to be published in 1996.

Following the Directorate of Health Care's recent assumption of responsibility for the development of policy about occupational health and safety within Prison Service establishments, a revised Prison Service Health and Safety Policy Statement was issued, which reflected the status of the Service as an Executive Agency. Two new health care standards - on clinical services for drug misusers and the use of medicines - were issued to all prison establishments by the Directorate of Health Care.

The report of a review of HIV/AIDS in prison by the AIDS Advisory Committee, which contained 39 recommendations aimed at the development of a strategic approach to HIV infection, was published[4], as was the report of the first national survey of the physical health of male sentenced prisoners[5]. This OPCS report showed ample evidence of high-risk behaviour among sentenced male prisoners - such as smoking cigarettes, and alcohol and drugs misuse before entry into prison - although standards of physical fitness were generally good.

Policy development towards designation as a World Health Organization (WHO) collaborating centre for health promoting prisons continued. A Working Group met in London to examine the feasibility of this initiative being based within the Directorate of Health Care of HM Prison Service.

References

1. HM Prison Service. *Drug misuse in prison.* London: HM Prison Service, 1995.
2. Lord President's Office. *Tackling drugs together: a strategy for England: 1995-1998.* London: HMSO, 1995 (Cm. 2846).
3. *The Mental Health Act 1983.* London: HMSO, 1983.
4. HM Prison Service. *The Review of HIV/AIDS in prison by the AIDS Advisory Committee, HM Prison Service: England and Wales.* London: HM Prison Service, 1995.
5. Bridgewood A, Malbon G. *Survey of the physical health of prisoners: 1994.* London: HMSO, 1995.

CHAPTER 6

COMMUNICABLE DISEASES

(a)   HIV infection and AIDS

Government strategy on HIV infection and AIDS

A strategy group reviewed HIV and AIDS health promotion and its report, *An evolving strategy*, was published in November[1]. This revised and more focused health promotion strategy:

— places greater emphasis on appropriate targeting of high-risk groups (ie, homosexual and bisexual men, people with links to high-prevalence countries, injecting drug misusers and female partners of men from these groups);

— recognises that some national HIV/AIDS campaigns are needed to maintain public awareness;

— recognises that community-based and self-help organisations are well placed to develop targeted health promotion work; *and*

— highlights the need for commissioning authorities to use a variety of approaches and to evaluate outcomes, and for areas of low prevalence to take particular care to avoid complacency.

Progress of the epidemic

AIDS

Surveillance of the epidemic is implemented through the voluntary confidential reporting systems run by the Public Health Laboratory Service (PHLS) AIDS Centre[2,3] and the Government's programme of unlinked anonymous HIV surveys[4].

Details of the AIDS cases reported in England are shown in Table 6.1 and Figure 6.1; 1,418 cases of AIDS were reported in 1995: these brought the cumulative total of AIDS cases reported since 1982 to 10,915, of whom 7,477 are known to have died. It is estimated that, on average, people newly diagnosed with AIDS were infected with HIV some 10 years previously.

Figure 6.2 compares the incidence rates of AIDS diagnoses per million population of various European countries for 1995 (previous Reports showed cumulative rates, not incidence rates).

HIV infection

Table 6.2 and Figure 6.3 show details of reports of the 2,485 people with newly diagnosed HIV infection in England, bringing the cumulative total of such

Table 6.1: *AIDS cases and known deaths by exposure category and date of report, England, 1982-31 December 1995*
(Numbers subject to revision as further data are received or duplicates identified)

How persons probably acquired the virus	Jan 1994-Dec 1994		Jan 1995-Dec 1995		Jan 1982-Dec 1995			
	Cases		Cases		Male		Female	
	Male	Female	Male	Female	Cases	Deaths	Cases	Deaths
Sexual intercourse								
Between men	1089	-	914	-	7995	5659	-	-
Between men and women								
Exposure to 'high risk' partner*	6	15	3	23	34	20	107	67
Exposure abroad**	136	96	111	111	661	370	487	245
Exposure in UK	14	15	8	7	65	42	55	37
Investigation continuing/closed†	5	-	13	4	21	3	4	-
Injecting drug use (IDU)	67	27	49	19	303	182	131	71
IDU and sexual intercourse								
between men	28	-	18	-	182	126	-	-
Blood								
Blood factor								
(eg treatment for haemophilia)	65	-	80	-	487	428	5	4
Blood/tissue transfer								
(eg transfusion)								
Abroad	2	2	2	1	14	7	41	24
UK	2	3	2	2	21	15	23	18
Mother to infant	22	22	16	17	83	44	85	39
Other/undetermined	10	1	10	8	92	67	19	9
Total	1446	181	1226	192	9958	6963	957	514

* Partner(s) exposed to HIV infection through sexual intercourse between men, injecting drug users, or those infected through blood factor treatment or blood/tissue transfer.

** Individuals from abroad and individuals from the UK who have lived or visited abroad, for whom there is no evidence of 'high risk' partners.

† Closed = no further information available.

Source: CDSC. PHLS

Figure 6.1: *AIDS cases: total numbers and numbers where infection was probably acquired through sexual intercourse between men and women, England, to 31 December 1995*

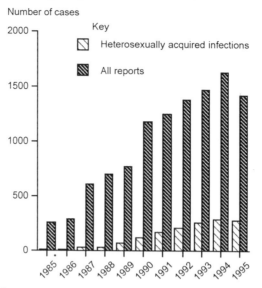

Number of cases

Key
⬚ Heterosexually acquired infections
▨ All reports

* 1985 or earlier

Source: CDSC, PHLS

Figure 6.2: *Incidence of AIDS cases diagnosed in Europe in 1995, adjusted for reporting delays: rates per million population*

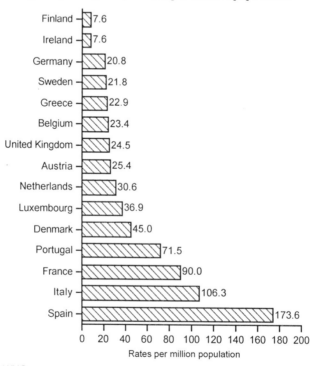

Country	Rate
Finland	7.6
Ireland	7.6
Germany	20.8
Sweden	21.8
Greece	22.9
Belgium	23.4
United Kingdom	24.5
Austria	25.4
Netherlands	30.6
Luxembourg	36.9
Denmark	45.0
Portugal	71.5
France	90.0
Italy	106.3
Spain	173.6

Rates per million population

Source: WHO

Table 6.2: *HIV-1 infected persons by exposure category and date of report, England, to 31 December 1995*
(Numbers subject to revision as further data are received or duplicates identified)

How persons probably acquired the virus	Jan 1994-Dec 1994			Jan 1995-Dec 1995			Nov 1984-Dec 1995		
	Male	Female	NK†	Male	Female	NK†	Male	Female	NK†
Sexual intercourse									
Between men	1252	-	-	1304	-	-	14272	-	-
Between men and women									
Exposure to 'high risk' partner*	7	31	-	11	36	-	74	364	-
Exposure abroad**	240	261	1	277	290	2	1652	1584	7
Exposure in the UK	21	29	-	20	25	-	114	187	-
Investigation continuing/closed‡	10	17	-	53	54	1	86	93	1
Injecting drug use (IDU)	108	50	-	109	43	2	1193	539	5
IDU and sexual intercourse									
between men	29	-	-	25	-	-	335	-	-
Blood									
Blood factor treatment									
(eg for haemophilia)	4	-	-	10	-	-	1073	10	-
Blood/tissue transfer									
(eg transfusion)									
Abroad/UK	5	8	-	2	7	-	62	73	3
Mother to infant‡	36	29	1	13	15	1	153	152	2
Other/undetermined/closed¶	56	13	-	143	37	5	623	112	36
Total	1768	438	2	1967	507	11	19637	3114	54

† NK = Not known (sex not stated on report).
* Partner(s) exposed to HIV infection through sexual intercourse between men, with injecting drug users, or with those infected through blood factor treatment or blood/tissue transfer.
** Individuals from abroad, and individuals from the UK who have lived or visited abroad, for whom there is no evidence of 'high risk' partners.
‡ By date of report that established infected status of infant.
¶ Closed = no further information available.

Source: CDSC, PHLS

Figure 6.3: *HIV antibody-positive people: total numbers and numbers where infection was probably acquired through sexual intercourse between men and women, England, by year of report to 31 December 1995*

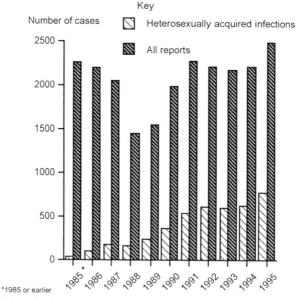

Source: CDSC, PHLS

reports since 1984 to 22,805. However, many factors might influence the decision to be tested for HIV infection, and these figures underestimate the true cumulative number of HIV infections.

Unlinked anonymous surveillance

The second report from the Government's Unlinked Anonymous HIV Surveys Steering Group[4] was published in December. These surveys were set up in January 1990 to supplement data from voluntary confidential testing and to permit a more accurate picture of the epidemic. The surveys are established in a number of genito-urinary medicine (GUM) clinics, centres for injecting drug misusers and antenatal clinics; screening of dried blood spots from neonates also takes place.

Results are summarised in Table 6.3 and show that, whilst prevalence is highest in London, HIV-1 infection is present in high-risk groups in every region surveyed. The prevalence rate in 1994 among homosexual or bisexual men attending GUM clinics was 11.3% in London and the South-East compared with 3.4% elsewhere.

Prevalence rates among injecting drug users (IDUs) were 3.0% for men and 4.0% for women in London and the South-East, and less than 1% in men and women alike elsewhere. This group remain vulnerable because about one-fifth of current IDUs report sharing of injecting equipment, with young injectors and women reporting significantly higher rates of sharing.

Table 6.3: Prevalence of HIV-1 infection in the unlinked anonymous survey groups, England and Wales, 1994

Survey group	London and South-East England*				England and Wales outside South-East England				Prevalence ratio‡ London vs elsewhere
	Number tested	Number HIV-1 infected	% HIV-1 infected	Prevalence range (%)†	Number tested	Number HIV-1 infected	% HIV-1 infected	Prevalence range (%)†	
Males									
Genito-urinary medicine clinic attenders									
Homo/bisexual§	3733	423	11.33	3.10, 21.92	1417	48	3.38	1.40, 4.50	4.0
Heterosexual§	11713	105	0.90	0.31, 2.12	16027	22	0.14	0, 0.36	7.5
Injecting drug users attending agencies#	604	18	3.0	1.3, 5.9	1912	6	0.3	0, 0.7	9.5
Hospital blood counts (sentinel group)	13003	78	0.60	0.30, 0.94	-	-	-	-	-
Females									
Genito-urinary medicine clinic attenders									
Heterosexual§	15691	75	0.48	0.12, 0.80	14575	6	0.04	0, 0.14	11.6
Injecting drug users attending agencies#	224	9	4.0	1.6, 7.4	643	4	0.6	0, 3.7	6.5
Pregnant women at delivery (infant dried blood spots)**	105097	180	0.17	0, 0.47	268652	28	0.01	0, 0.27	13.9
Pregnant women seeking terminations	8665	54	0.62	0.26, 1.01	-	-	-	-	-
Hospital blood counts (sentinel group)	26193	51	0.19	0.05, 0.27	-	-	-	-	-

* The injecting drug user (IDU) survey includes data from a few agencies in the South-East outside London; all other surveys present data for London.

† The range within a category is the lowest and highest rates recorded in individual genito-urinary medicine clinics (GUM survey), districts (infant dried blood spot survey) or hospitals (termination of pregnancy and antenatal surveys).

§ Excluding known drug users.

Attending specialist centres for IDUs.

** Prevalence in South-East England outside London was 0.02% (16 of 81,263) in 1993. In Northern and Yorkshire Region data for pregnant women come from the antenatal survey.

‡ The ratio by which the prevalence of infection in London is greater than the prevalence in England and Wales outside South-East England.

Source: Unlinked Anonymous HIV Surveys

161

Figure 6.4: *Trends in prevalence of HIV-1 infection among pregnant women by area of residence, Thames health Regions, 1988-94*

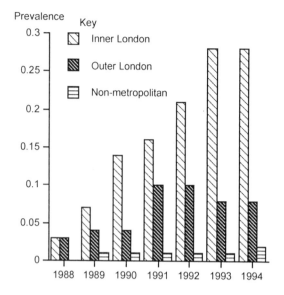

Source: Survey in North Thames and South Thames (West) co-ordinated by Institute of Child Health, London; survey elsewhere co-ordinated by PHLS AIDS Centre (commenced in 1990)

Table 6.4: *HIV in blood donations in the United Kingdom, October 1985 to December 1995*

Year	Donations tested (million)	Donations confirmed HIV-seropositive			
		Male	Female	Total	%
1985	0.6	13	0	13	0.002
1986	2.64	44	9	53	0.002
1987	2.59	18	5	23	0.0009
1988	2.64	18*	5	23*	0.0009
1989	2.74	25	12	37	0.001
1990	2.82	20*†	12	32*†	0.001
1991	2.95	23	8	31	0.001
1992	2.90	15	11	26	0.0009
1993	2.92	16	4	20	0.0007
1994	2.91	8	8	16	0.0005
1995	2.90	20	10	30	0.001
Total	*28.61*	*220*	*84*	*304*	*0.001*

*Updated figures.
†Includes one anti-HIV-2-positive donation.

Source: National Blood Authority

In London, HIV-1 prevalence among pregnant women in 1994 was 1 in 580 (see Figure 6.4). Comparison of data from the surveys with reported births to HIV-1 infected mothers indicate that only 17% of these infections have been clinically recognised. Outside London and the South-East, prevalence among pregnant women was 1 in 9,600 - one-fourteenth of that in London, but higher than in 1993.

HIV/AIDS projections

A summary of a report on AIDS projections for England and Wales until 1999 was published in November[5]. At the end of 1999, it is projected that there will be about 4,000 people with AIDS alive in the population, and about an additional 4,000 people with other forms of severe HIV disease. The overall incidence of AIDS cases is expected to level off in 1996 and 1997. AIDS incidence among homosexual males may fall, whereas the incidence among those exposed heterosexually or by intravenous drug misuse is expected to increase gradually. It is estimated that at the end of 1993 there were 21,900 adults infected with HIV in England and Wales[4].

AIDS/HIV infected health care workers

The Working Group to review the risk of HIV transmission from infected health care workers to patients reported to the United Kingdom (UK) Advisory Panel for Health Care Workers Infected with Bloodborne Viruses. Cases are considered individually by the Panel in light of the report's conclusion that a small number of surgical procedures may pose a small rather than extremely remote risk of HIV transmission from an infected health care worker to a patient.

HIV in blood donations

During 1995, 2.9 million blood donations in the UK were tested with anti-HIV-1+2 combined tests. Thirty donations (from 20 males and 10 females) were found to be anti-HIV-1 seropositive, or 1 in 96,700 (0.001%). The number of new donors tested were 352,000, of whom 17 were seropositive (1 in 20,705, or 0.005%). Again, no donations were found to be anti-HIV-2 seropositive during 1995.

Table 6.4 shows the number of donations tested in the UK between the Autumn of 1985 and the end of 1995, together with the number of donations confirmed as HIV seropositive. The male:female ratio of seropositive donations in 1995 was 2 to 1, and was 1.8 to 1 for new donors.

Public education and prevention

The Health Education Authority (HEA) continued to produce information, including radio and press campaigns, about HIV transmission and other sexually transmitted diseases (STDs).

The new integrated national AIDS/Drugs Helpline began on 1 April, although the services remain distinct. This telephone helpline continues to play a valuable role in the Government's HIV strategy.

References

1. UK Health Departments. *HIV & AIDS health promotion: an evolving strategy.* London: Department of Health, 1995.
2. Public Health Laboratory Service AIDS Centre. The surveillance of HIV-1 infection and AIDS in England and Wales. *Commun Dis Rep* 1991; **1**: R51-R56.
3. Wight PA, Rush AM, Miller E. Surveillance of HIV infection by voluntary testing in England. *Commun Dis Rep* 1992; **2**: R85-R90.
4. Unlinked Anonymous HIV Surveys Steering Group. *Unlinked anonymous HIV prevalence monitoring programme: England and Wales: data to the end of 1994.* London: Department of Health, 1995.
5. Public Health Laboratory Service. The incidence and prevalence of AIDS and prevalence of other severe HIV disease in England and Wales for 1995 to 1999: projections using data to the end of 1994: report of an Expert Group convened by the Director of the Public Health Laboratory Service on behalf of the Chief Medical Officers. *Commun Dis Rev* 1995; **6(1)**: R1-R24.

(b)   Other sexually transmitted diseases

The total number of new cases seen in GUM clinics in England continued to rise, with 722,565 seen in 1994, an increase of 9% over 1993 (see Table 6.5); these figures represent a rise of 6% among men and 12% in women. STDs and other infections requiring treatment were diagnosed in 53% overall (in 49% of men and 56% of women). Numbers of patients for whom no treatment was required or referral elsewhere was indicated also continued to rise. Overall, the number of reports of confirmed STDs and other infections rose by 8% from 353,752 to 381,025. Of these, approximately 23% were for wart virus infection, 17% for non-specific genital infection, 10% for *Chlamydia*, 7% for herpes simplex virus (HSV), 3% for gonorrhoea and 2% for pelvic inflammatory disease (PID). All figures are derived from the KC60 reporting form for consultations in NHS GUM clinics; cases diagnosed and managed without reference to GUM clinics are therefore not included. The comparisons below are with previous KC60 data.

In 1994, total reports of gonorrhoea fell by 2% compared with 1993, from 11,803 to 11,574 (a decrease of less than 1% in men and of 4% in women). This is equivalent to a rate of 37 per 100,000 population in 1994 (see Figure 6.5). The Health of the Nation target[1] is to reduce the incidence of gonorrhoea among men and women aged 15-64 years by at least 20% by 1995, or a reduction from the 1990 rate of 61 cases per 100,000 population to no more than 49 cases per 100,000. This target was achieved in 1992, when the rate fell to 45 cases per 100,000 population.

The total number of reports of uncomplicated chlamydial infection rose by 9% to 36,097 (an increase of 8% in men and 9% in women). Uncomplicated non-specific genital infections rose by 10% from 60,110 in 1993 to 65,974 in 1994. There was a rise of 22% in reports of PID among women, from 6,295 in 1993 to 7,690 in 1994.

164

Table 6.5: *Sexually transmitted diseases, and other infections that may be sexually transmitted, reported by NHS genito-urinary medicine clinics, England, in year ending 31 December 1994*

Condition	Males	Females	Persons
All syphilis	883	510	1393
Infectious syphilis	*194*	*110*	*304*
All gonorrhoea (excluding PID and epididymitis)	7273	4301	11574
Post-pubertal uncomplicated	*6431*	*3201*	*9632*
All *Chlamydia* (excluding PID and chlamydial infections with arthritis)[1]	16977	19120	36097
Post-pubertal uncomplicated chlamydia	*12449*	*15125*	*27574*
Pelvic infection and epididymitis	1524	7690	9214
Non-specific urethritis (NSU) and related disease	48389	17585	65974
Chlamydial infections/NSU with arthritis	309	125	434
Chancroid/Donovanosis/LGV	40	22	62
Trichomoniasis	323	5236	5559
Vaginosis/vaginitis/balanitis	12160	41734	53894
Candidiasis	9248	55539	64787
Scabies/pediculosis	3848	1203	5051
All Herpes simplex	11906	14899	26805
Herpes simplex-first attack	*6255*	*9092*	*15347*
Herpes simplex-recurrence	*5651*	*5807*	*11458*
All Wart virus infection	49694	37031	86725
Wart virus infection-first attack	*25467*	*23585*	*49052*
Wart virus infection-recurrence	*24227*	*13446*	*37673*
Viral hepatitis	810	274	1084
Asymptomatic HIV infection - first presentation	1055	288	1343
Asymptomatic HIV infection - subsequent presentation	*8549*	*1302*	*9851*
HIV infection with symptoms, not AIDS - first presentation	1366	202	1568
AIDS - first presentation	1089	126	1215
Other conditions requiring treatment[2]	69577	68197	137774
Other episodes not requiring treatment	101873	95554	197427
Other conditions referred elsewhere	6767	7818	14585
Total number of new cases seen	345111	377454	722565

[1]   Comprises 'uncomplicated chlamydial infection', 'other complicated chlamydia (excluding PID and epididymitis)' and 'Chlamydia ophthalmia neonatorum'.

[2]   Includes epidemiological treatment of trichomoniasis, vaginosis, vaginitis, balanitis and candidiasis.

LGV = lymphogranuloma venereum; PID = pelvic inflammatory disease.

Source: Form KC60

Figure 6.5: *All gonorrhoea: number of new cases seen at NHS genito-urinary medicine clinics, England, 1980-94*

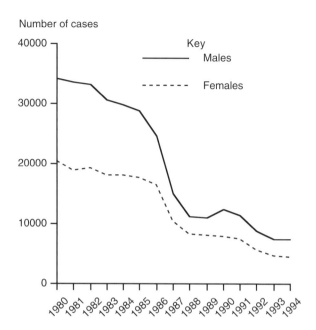

Source: Forms SBH60 and KC60

There was a small increase in reports of syphilis (3%), due to an increase of 15% for non-infectious syphilis in women, and a small decrease in reports of infectious syphilis (304 cases in 1994 compared with 337 in 1993).

First attacks of HSV infection remained virtually the same in men at 6,255 cases and rose by approximately 9% in women to 9,092 cases, an overall rise of 5%. First attacks of HSV are more common in women, accounting for 59% of such reports. Recurrent attacks rose by 5% in men and 6% in women, and accounted for 43% of all reports of HSV infection during 1994.

Total reports of viral warts rose by 2%, and recurrent attacks accounted for 43% of all reports of wart virus infection during 1994.

A high proportion of reports of STDs come from patients in younger age-groups (see Table 6.6).

Reference

1. Department of Health. *The Health of the Nation: a strategy for health in England.* London: HMSO, 1992 (Cm. 1986).

Table 6.6: *New cases of selected conditions reported by NHS genito-urinary medicine clinics by age (in years), England, 1994*

Condition	Sex	All ages	Under 16	16-19	20-24	25-34	35-44	45 and over	Estimated median age
Infectious syphilis	M	194	0	2	34	79	47	32	32
	F	110	2	5	37	45	11	10	27
Post-pubertal uncomplicated gonorrhoea	M	6431	36	652	1724	3026	718	275	27
	F	3201	77	989	1095	850	154	36	22
Post-pubertal uncomplicated *Chlamydia*	M	12449	49	1092	4294	5470	1128	416	26
	F	15125	300	4179	5812	4048	638	148	22
Herpes simplex - first attack	M	6255	16	339	1415	2888	1038	559	29
	F	9092	109	1523	2891	3242	924	403	25
Wart virus infection - first attack	M	25467	89	1786	8958	10673	2712	1249	26
	F	23585	381	5826	8897	6155	1581	745	23

Source: Form KC60

167

(c)   Immunisation

Immunisation coverage

Coverage for most of the routinely provided childhood vaccines has continued to rise. For vaccines against diphtheria, tetanus, polio and *Haemophilus influenzae* type b (Hib), coverage by the second birthday is 95% (see Appendix Table A.9). For these antigens, national vaccination coverage targets have been met. There has been slight slippage of coverage for measles, mumps, rubella (MMR) vaccine, down 1% to 91%; this fall may be related to the publicity about adverse events that accompanied the November 1994 measles, rubella immunisation campaign, although the frequency of such events was very low (only one in 6,700 children in the UK experienced any adverse reaction, and only one in 15,000 had a reaction categorised as 'serious')[1,2]. Collection of all immunisation coverage statistics is now on a UK-wide basis, with quarterly data provided through computerised systems by all four Health Departments using consistent numerators and denominators. The number of cases of diphtheria, tetanus, pertussis and Hib remain extremely low; there have been no cases of wild virus poliomyelitis.

Measles, rubella immunisation campaign

The full impact of the 1994 measles, rubella immunisation campaign is now apparent. During 1995, measles cases have been exceptionally rare; most of those cases that were confirmed occurred either in unimmunised children under the age for routine immunisation, or in those who were too young or too old to have been included in the school-based campaign. In a number of confirmed cases, there was evidence that they had been imported from West Africa, Asia or neighbouring European countries. These encouraging findings should be seen against predictions of a measles epidemic in 1995/96; notifications in 1994 had been rising in line with those seen in 1987, shortly before the 1988 measles epidemic[3,4] (see Figure 6.6).

Since November 1994, notified cases of suspected measles have been investigated by examination of saliva for measles-(and rubella)-specific IgM. Approximately 50-60% of notified cases were investigated in this way, and only 1% of notified cases were confirmed to be measles infections (see Figure 6.7).

Serological surveillance has demonstrated the impact of the immunisation campaign[4]. After the campaign there was a considerable decline in susceptibility for both measles and rubella in the age-group immunised in November 1994. The proportion of 5-16-year-olds who were antibody-negative for measles fell from 10.3% in 1994 to 3% in 1995. For rubella, the corresponding decline in males aged 5-16 years was from 20.1% to 6.1%; for females in this age-group, the rate was from 10.5% to 1.8% (from PHLS data), which confirms the importance of including rubella immunisation in the vaccination programme. As a consequence of this finding, and the maintenance of high MMR coverage by the second birthday since that vaccine's introduction in 1988, the schoolgirl rubella immunisation programme has now been stopped. To consolidate these

Figure 6.6: *Numbers of measles notifications, England and Wales, 1987-89 and 1994-96*

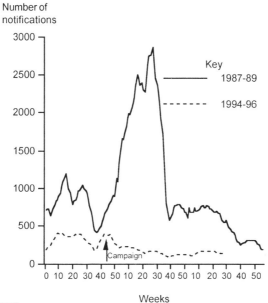

Source: OPCS/ONS

Figure 6.7: *Measles surveillance: notifications, saliva tests and confirmed positive cases, England and Wales, 1994-96*

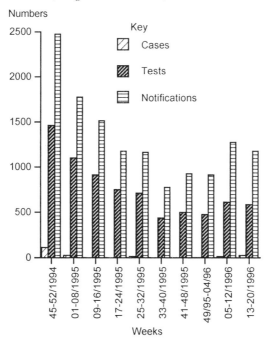

Source: PHLS

169

gains in measles and rubella control, and to prevent the re-accumulation of a pool of susceptible individuals sufficient to allow for future epidemics, a second dose of MMR vaccine has been recommended to be given to all children at the same time as the pre-school booster of diphtheria, tetanus and polio vaccines.

References

1. Committee on Safety of Medicines, Medicines Control Agency. Adverse reactions to measles/rubella vaccine. *Curr Probl Pharmacovigilance* 1995; **21:** 9-10.
2. Department of Health. Measles, rubella (MR) immunisation campaign 1994: one year on. *CMO's Update* 1995; **8:** 1.
3. Department of Health. *National measles and rubella immunisation campaign.* London: Department of Health, 1994 (Professional Letter: PL/CMO (94)10).
4. Department of Health. *On the State of the Public Health: the annual report of the Chief Medical Officer of the Department of Health for the year 1994.* London: HMSO, 1995; 171-9.

(d)   Viral hepatitis

Acute viral hepatitis is a notifiable disease. In 1995, a provisional total of 3,156 cases were notified to the Office of Population Censuses and Surveys (OPCS, to become part of the Office for National Statistics [ONS] in 1996) for England. Of these, 2,043 were due to hepatitis A and 599 to hepatitis B. A further source of data is obtained through the voluntary confidential reporting by laboratories of confirmed cases to PHLS CDSC.

Hepatitis A

The incidence of hepatitis A infections fluctuates, the most recent peak being in 1990 when 7,248 cases were reported to the CDSC for England. Reports have decreased in each of the five successive years, with 1,689 reports being received in 1995 (see Figure 6.8). Most cases of hepatitis A infection seen in England are acquired in the UK and while most of these are sporadic, outbreaks do occur. However, a history of travel abroad in the six weeks before the onset of illness was recorded in 220 (13%) of cases reported to the CDSC in 1995 (see page 182).

Hepatitis B

Reports of acute hepatitis B peaked in 1984 in England and subsequently fell (see Figure 6.9). The CDSC received reports of 584 cases in 1995, and information about risk exposure was available in 373 (64%). Where such information was available, 19% were likely to have acquired infection as a result of sexual intercourse between men, 25% as a result of sexual intercourse between men and women and 36% as a result of intravenous drug misuse. Much acute hepatitis B is subclinical, not diagnosed and hence not reported.

Hepatitis C

Each donation of blood is tested for antibodies to HIV-1, HIV-2, hepatitis B surface antigen and hepatitis C. Precise figures for hepatitis C are difficult to provide for the calendar year due to delays caused by confirmatory testing. However, the frequency of confirmed positive results is 20-30 times more

Figure 6.8: *Reports of hepatitis A to CDSC, England, 1980-95*

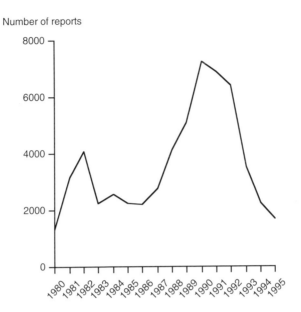

Source: PHLS, CDSC

Figure 6.9: *Reports of hepatitis B to CDSC (all reports and reports in injecting drug users), England, 1980-95*

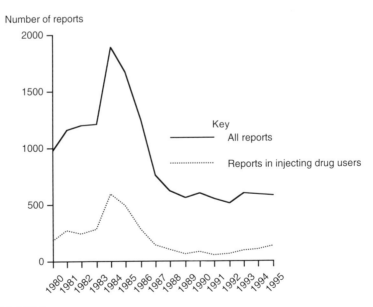

Source: PHLS, CDSC

common among new donors than in established donors. (Figures vary from 1 in 1,200 to 1 in 2,000 for new donors, and from 1 in 23,000 to 1 in 66,000 for established donors for different months or quarters of the year.)

Possible novel hepatitis virus

Two independent research teams have recently used molecular virological techniques to describe viruses derived from the sera of different individual patients with hepatitis, which have been provisionally designated the hepatitis GB agent (GBV) (GB being the initials of the patient from whose serum this agent was originally derived)[1,2] and 'hepatitis G virus' (HGV)[3]. Three GBV agents have been cloned, suffixed A,B and C: only GBV-C appears to be a human virus. The molecular sequences of HGV and GBV-C are more than 90% homologous; it would appear that HGV and GBV-C are independent isolates of the same virus (a member of the *Flaviviridae* family, but distinct from hepatitis C).

The prevalence of HGV/GBV-C among voluntary blood donors in the United States of America is around 1.6%, and hence it is more prevalent in that population than hepatitis C. HGV/GBV-C has been shown to have been transmitted by blood transfusion and a higher prevalence has been found among people with frequent parenteral exposure - such as intravenous drug users, haemophiliacs, patients treated by maintenance haemodialysis and those who have received multiple transfusions. It has been found in some patients with acute and chronic hepatitis, but to what extent it may cause acute liver injury or lead to serious chronic liver disease remains uncertain. The full clinical significance of HGV/GBV-C infection and of its natural history are unknown and require further study, which should also help to define whether it is a true hepatotropic virus.

References

1. Simons JN, Leary TP, Dawson GJ et al. Isolation of novel virus-like sequences associated with human hepatitis. *Nature Med* 1995; **1:** 564-9.
2. Leary TP, Muerhoff AS, Simons JN et al. Sequence and genomic organisation of GBV-C: a novel member of the *Flaviviridae* associated with human non-A-E hepatitis. *J Med Virol* (in press).
3. Linnen J, Wages J Jr, Zhang-Keck ZY et al. Molecular cloning and disease association of hepatitis G virus: a transfusion transmissible agent. *Science* (in press).

(e) Influenza

Two peaks of influenza activity occurred during 1995 (see Figure 6.10). The peak for the Winter of 1994/95 was in February 1995, with weekly general practitioner (GP) consultation rates for new episodes of influenza-like illness reaching 159 per 100,000 population, mostly due to influenza B. By contrast, the influenza season for 1995/96 started early, with weekly GP consultation rates reaching a peak of 176 per 100,000 population in the first week of December. The commonest strains were influenza A (H_3N_2) viruses similar to those which had been expected, and were covered by the vaccine. A review of past data indicates that during a normal Winter, weekly GP consultation rates for new episodes of influenza-like illness can be expected to reach levels of up to 150-200 per 100,000 population, whereas in severe epidemics they always exceed 400 per 100,000 population weekly. By these criteria, the peaks for both 1994/95 and 1995/96 could be considered at the upper end of the expected normal Winter increase, although at the time the 1995/96 increase was considered a 'moderate' epidemic.

GPs were reminded in July of current influenza immunisation policy and advised to plan their immunisation programmes and order their vaccine supplies early[1]; the subsequent annual influenza immunisation letter in September confirmed which vaccines were available[2]. Over 6 million doses of influenza vaccine were distributed and no shortages occurred. DH produced a patient information leaflet *What should I do about 'flu?*[3], which contained advice about how to recognise, and what to do about, influenzal illness. The leaflet proved popular and, in the light of consumer research, will be re-issued in a slightly modified version, together with a further leaflet about influenza immunisation.

Major epidemics and pandemics of influenza are unpredictable. The Department has therefore continued to evolve contingency plans for an influenza pandemic. These will be presented to Ministers and are expected to be published in 1996. The plans will be kept under review so that they keep abreast of new developments and organisational arrangements.

Figure 6.10: *General practice consultation rates for influenza-like illness, England and Wales, 1994-95 and 1995-96*

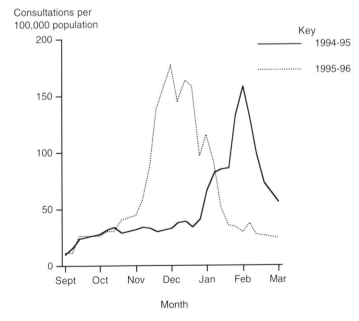

Source: RCGP weekly returns

References

1. Department of Health. Influenza immunisation. *CMO's Update* 1995; **6**: 4.
2. Department of Health. *Influenza immunisation.* Wetherby (West Yorkshire): Department of Health, 1995 (Professional Letter: PL/CMO(95)2).
3. Department of Health. *What should I do about 'flu?* Wetherby (West Yorkshire): Department of Health, 1995.

(f)   Meningitis

Notifications and laboratory isolates of meningococci rose considerably in 1995 to reach levels not seen since 1989/90. The seasonal rise occurred earlier than usual, the overall number of cases increased, and an upward shift in the age distribution of cases was noted (see Figure 6.11). There was a shift towards more Group C meningococcal infections (from less than 30% of isolations in early 1995 to more than 40% by the end of the year), and more cases with septicaemic features at presentation. Despite this increase in septicaemia, overall case-fatality rates have fallen from 58% in 1989 to 20% in 1995. More cases with clinical presentations compatible with meningococcal infection are culture negative than in the past, which may reflect increasing use of pre-admission penicillin, which in turn may be contributing to the reduced case fatality[1,2]. However, the increasing availability of molecular diagnostic techniques now enables identification of meningococcal infection in suspected cases that are culture negative[3].

Figure 6.11: *Cases of meningococcal disease, England and Wales, 1989-95*

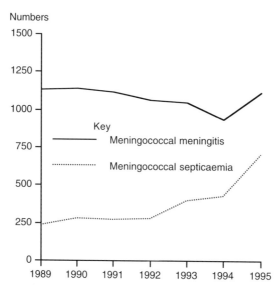

Source: PHLS

174

In the course of the 1995 upsurge of meningococcal infections, there were a number of clusters of cases where no epidemiological links could be found other than attendance at the same school. When these outbreaks involved Group C meningococci, immunisation of whole schools was carried out with Group C meningococcal polysaccharide vaccine. In three local outbreaks, no links between cases could be identified, and all young people in those areas aged 2-20 years were offered vaccine. In the three Districts/NHS Trusts where such widespread immunisation was performed, no further cases were reported. Nevertheless, presently available meningococcal vaccines are unsuitable for routine application as they are not immunogenic in children aged under 2 years, who are the group at highest risk, and the duration of protection is short lived. DH is sponsoring trials of new Group C conjugated vaccines for use at 2, 3 and 4 months along with other routinely administered vaccines; a Group B vaccine is also being evaluated as a collaboration between the Department of Health, CDSC and Rijksinstituut voor Volksgezondheid en Milieuhygiene (RIVM), the Dutch national vaccine manufacturer.

References

1. Research Committee of the British Society for the Study of Infections. Bacterial meningitis: causes for concern. Special report. *J Infection* 1995; **30**: 84-94.
2. Department of Health. Meningococcal infection. *CMO's Update* 1995; **7**: 2.
3. Public Health Laboratory Service. Polymerase chain reaction for diagnosis of meningococcal infection. *CDR Weekly* 1995; **5(33)**: 155.

(g)   Tuberculosis

Data for 1995 indicate that notifications of tuberculosis have levelled out following the small year-on-year increases seen between 1991 and 1993. A total of 5,608 cases were notified in England and Wales in 1995, compared with 5,591 in 1994 and 5,961 in 1993.

Undernotification of tuberculosis, particularly in patients with HIV infection, has been well documented. In April, the Department reminded doctors of their statutory duty to notify all cases of tuberculosis[1]. The main purpose of notification is to ensure that contact-tracing procedures are instituted. Failure to notify may result in failure to detect associated cases or to manage contacts correctly.

In December, consultants in communicable disease control (CsCDC) published a report on tuberculosis in London, which accounted for 38% of all notifications in England and Wales in 1994[2]. Several studies looked in more detail at the known risk-factors for tuberculosis in London. In one East London district, ethnic mix alone did not appear to account for the whole of the observed increase in cases, an increase also being seen in the white population[3], but while higher rates of tuberculosis have long been recognised to occur in poorer inner-city areas, another study found that separating the various indicators of socio-economic deprivation was very difficult[4]. A study among users of open-access hostels for the homeless confirmed a high incidence of tuberculosis, particularly among older men with a history of alcohol misuse[5].

Drug-resistant tuberculosis has remained at low levels, but the first UK nosocomial outbreak of multidrug-resistant tuberculosis, in an HIV unit in London, was reported in August[6].

The Inter-Departmental Working Group on Tuberculosis consulted widely over its recommendations to improve measures for the prevention and control of tuberculosis in the UK and completed its first two reports[7,8]. A further expert working group was established to make recommendations for the prevention and control of HIV-related and drug-resistant tuberculosis, and is expected to report during 1996.

References

1. Department of Health. *Notification of tuberculosis in patients with HIV infection.* Wetherby (West Yorkshire): Department of Health, 1995.
2. The London Consultants in Communicable Disease Control Group. *The surveillance, prevention and control of tuberculosis in London.* London: United Medical Schools of Guy's and St Thomas's Hospitals, 1995.
3. Bhatti N, Law MR, Morris JK, Halliday R, Moore Gillon J. Increasing incidence of tuberculosis in England and Wales: a study of the likely causes. *BMJ* 1995; **310**: 967-9.
4. Mangtani P, Jolley DJ, Watson JM, Rodrigues LC. Socio-economic deprivation and notification rates for tuberculosis in London during 1982-91. *BMJ* 1995; **310**: 963-6.
5. Citron KM, Southern A, Dixon M. *Out of the shadows.* London: Crisis, 1995.
6. Communicable Disease Surveillance Centre. Outbreak of hospital-acquired multidrug-resistant tuberculosis. *Commun Dis Rep* 1995; **5**: 161.
7. Inter-Departmental Working Group on Tuberculosis. *Recommendations for the prevention and control of tuberculosis at local level.* London: UK Health Departments (in press).
8. Inter-Departmental Working Group on Tuberculosis. *Tuberculosis and homeless people.* London: UK Health Departments (in press).

(h)   Hospital-acquired infection

New guidance on hospital infection control, produced by a joint DH/PHLS working group chaired by Dr Mary Cooke, was issued in March[1]. It covers the role of the infection control team and committee, surveillance of hospital-acquired infection (HAI) and the management of outbreaks, and also provides information on the impact of HAI and advice to commissioners of health care. The guidance applies to NHS and independent hospitals alike, and has been well received.

Methicillin-resistant *Staphylococcus aureus* (MRSA) continued to be a problem in 1995, and PHLS received isolates from 190 hospitals that had incidents involving three or more patients who acquired the same strain. Most incidents involved the epidemic (EMRSA) strains 15 or 16, which spread particularly readily. Although most MRSA infections are relatively trivial and at least 80% of people with the organism have no evidence of infection, when serious conditions such as septicaemia or pneumonia arise they are difficult to treat.

Although the risk of people in the community developing MRSA infection is low, there has been increased anxiety among managers of residential and nursing homes about accepting people from hospital who may be carrying the organism.

176

Seminars for home managers, registration officers and insurers were held in the Autumn, and guidance will be issued during 1996.

Reference

1. Department of Health, Hospital Infection Working Group. *Hospital infection control: guidance on the control of infection in hospitals prepared by the Hospital Infection Working Group of the Department of Health and Public Health Laboratory Service.* Wetherby (West Yorkshire): Department of Health, 1995 (Health Service Guidelines: HSG (95)10).

(i)　　Foodborne and waterborne diseases

Foodborne diseases

The provisional number of cases of food poisoning (formally notified and ascertained by other means) in England and Wales reported to the OPCS in 1995 remained stable at 82,041 (see Table 6.7), compared with an actual total of 81,833 in 1994. This is the first time since 1991 that there has not been a marked upward trend. *Campylobacter* continues to be the micro-organism most commonly isolated from cases of human bacterial gastro-enteritis and the number of reports fell by 1% compared with 1994. The incidence of *Salmonella* infection was 2% less than in 1994. There was a 93% increase in the incidence of verocytotoxin-producing *Escherichia coli* (VTEC) serogroup O157. Listeriosis remains well below the level of the late 1980s.

Campylobacter enteritis

Campylobacter continues to be the most commonly isolated bacterium associated with acute gastro-enteritis in human beings. The provisional number of laboratory reports to CDSC of faecal isolations of *Campylobacter* in England and Wales fell slightly in 1995 to 43,902 (provisional) compared with the finalised total of 44,414 for 1994.

Salmonellosis

The number of isolates of *Salmonella* from human beings reported in England and Wales for 1995 and recorded on the PHLS Salmonella Data Set was 29,717, compared with 30,411 (corrected figure) in 1994 (see Table 6.8).

The commonest *Salmonella* to infect human beings in England and Wales continues to be *Salmonella enteritidis* phage type 4 (PT4), which is associated with poultry and eggs. In 1995, there were 12,351 cases reported, compared with 13,782 in 1994. The second most prevalent *Salmonella* to cause human salmonellosis is *Salmonella typhimurium* definitive type 104 (DT104). This bacterium can also infect a range of animals, especially cattle. During 1995, there were 3,698 human cases of *Salmonella typhimurium* DT104 infection, compared with 2,848 in 1994. About 80% of isolates are resistant to a number of antibiotics. The reason for the emergence of and increase in infection due to these multi-resistant micro-organisms is being investigated by DH, the Ministry of Agriculture, Fisheries and Food (MAFF) and the PHLS.

Table 6.7: *Food poisoning: reports to ONS, England and Wales, 1982-95*

Year	Total*
1982	14253
1983	17735
1984	20702
1985	19242
1986	23948
1987	29331
1988	39713
1989	52557
1990	52145
1991	52543
1992	63347
1993	68587
1994	81833**
1995	82041

* Statutorily notified to OPCS/ONS and ascertained by other means.
**Confirmed cases (not provisional as stated in last year's Report).

Source: OPCS/ONS

Verocytotoxin-producing Escherichia coli (VTEC)

During 1995, there were 792 isolations of VTEC O157 in England and Wales - a 93% increase compared with 1994. There was also an increase in the number of general outbreaks in 1995, and these accounted for at least 14% of the isolates of VTEC O157 (compared with only 3% in 1994). This increase in outbreaks, and improved ascertainment by clinical laboratories following publication of the report on VTEC by the Advisory Committee on the Microbiological Safety of Food (ACMSF)[1], have been contributory factors to the rise in reported isolations of VTEC O157 in 1995.

Following publication of this report, the Chief Medical Officer issued advice to groups vulnerable to infection such as children, pregnant women and elderly people not to consume unpasteurised milk from cows, sheep or goats[2]. A programme of research as recommended by the report is under consideration.

Listeria

There were 91 reported cases of human listeriosis in England and Wales during 1995, compared with 112 reports received by the PHLS in 1994. Only seven of the 91 cases were pregnancy-associated, the lowest figure so far recorded.

Advisory Committee on the Microbiological Safety of Food

The Committee published its report on VTEC in June[1]. The report made recommendations to protect public health, to fill gaps in knowledge and to assist in the development of prevention and control measures.

The Poultry Meat Working Group completed its review of poultry meat production and will publish its report early in 1996. Another working group has

Table 6.8: *Salmonella in human beings, England and Wales, January to December (inclusive), 1994 and 1995*

Serotype	1994*		1995†	
	Total cases	Imported cases	Total cases	Imported cases
S. enteritidis				
Phage type 4	13782	1245	12351	944
Other phage types	3589	699	3735	664
S. typhimurium				
Definitive type 104	2848	145	3698	125
Other definitive types	2674	319	2994	302
Other serotypes	7183	1742	6341	1373
Others untyped	335	58	598	112
Total	*30411*	*4208*	*29717*	*3520*

* 1994 data adjusted and finalised.
† 1995 data provisional.

Source: PHLS Salmonella Data Set

begun an extensive review of foodborne viral infections and is likely to report in 1997.

The Committee has also begun to examine the implications for food safety of the increased incidence of antibiotic-resistant foodborne pathogens in human beings and food animals.

Developments in food surveillance

In May, the Steering Group on the Microbiological Safety of Food was merged with the ACMSF. The ACMSF has now taken on responsibility for advising the Government on its microbiological food surveillance programme and relevant epidemiological trends, allowing greater integration between surveillance and advice.

A microbiological food surveillance group has been established to co-ordinate surveillance activities, and to identify through surveillance the need for action to ensure the microbiological safety of food. The group, which includes representatives from industry, universities and a research association, held its first meeting in November. In addition to reviewing current and future activities, the group will provide the ACMSF with suggestions for a food microbiological surveillance strategy.

During the year, the Department began to fund a survey of the microbiological status of raw cow's milk on retail sale in England and Wales. The results of this survey will inform policy on the microbiological safety of raw milk. DH also began funding surveys on *Salmonella* contamination in UK-produced eggs at retail outlets, and in imported eggs to see if there has been any change in prevalence since the surveys of 1991.

European Community (EC) Member States are required to participate in an annual sampling programme throughout the Community which is agreed by Member States and co-ordinated by the European Commission. The 1995 programme involved the sampling and examination of ready-to-eat salads and crudités on retail sale.

The major study of infectious intestinal disease (IID) in England will provide epidemiological information on routes of infection, including those involving foodstuffs. The study has progressed well, with microbiological work due to be completed by Spring, 1996. Epidemiological and microbiological results will then be analysed, with the final report expected in 1997.

The Food Safety (General Food Hygiene) Regulations 1995

The Food Safety (General Food Hygiene) Regulations 1995[3] came into force on 15 September. These Regulations contain important new requirements related to hazard analysis and staff hygiene training. Basic minimum hygiene standards are specified, but the Regulations are more risk-related than previous UK controls. As part of the implementation process, DH carried out a national training exercise on the Regulations for enforcers. A series of road shows were also held for food businesses.

It is hoped that the new legal framework, with its increased emphasis on operational practices and risk assessment, will provide a more effective approach to the prevention of foodborne illness.

Waterborne diseases

A large outbreak of cryptosporidiosis occurred in the South West during the Summer. A strong association with drinking water was reported[4].

Six other outbreaks of cryptosporidiosis were recorded. Two were associated with farm visits, and one with a paddling pool; no vehicle of infection was identified in a fourth. The other two outbreaks are still under investigation. One non-cryptosporidial outbreak was associated with a private supply of drinking water.

The second report of the Group of Experts on *Cryptosporidium* in Water Supplies was published in November[5]. The Group confirmed the importance of catchment control and optimisation of drinking water treatment in reducing the risk of waterborne cryptosporidiosis.

References

1. Advisory Committee on the Microbiological Safety of Food. *Report on verocytotoxin-producing Escherichia coli.* London: HMSO, 1995.
2. Department of Health. *Chief Medical Officer advises vulnerable groups to avoid raw milk.* London: Department of Health, 1995 (Press Release: H95/278).
3. *The Food Safety (General Food Hygiene) Regulations 1995.* London: HMSO, 1995 (Statutory Instrument: SI 1995 no. 1763).
4. Harrison S. *An outbreak of cryptosporidiosis in the South Devon area: August to September 1995.* Dartington (Devon): South and West Devon Health Commission, 1995.

5. Department of the Environment, Department of Health. *Cryptosporidium in water supplies: second report of the group of experts.* London: HMSO, 1995. Chair: Sir John Badenoch.

(j)   Emerging infectious diseases

As a result of growing international concern about the emergence of apparently new and the re-emergence of old human infectious diseases world wide, and about the need for international co-ordination of the response to such events, the World Health Organization (WHO) established on 1 October a new Division of Emerging and other Communicable Diseases Surveillance and Control to monitor and react to new events.

Incidents of particular concern during 1995 included an outbreak of Ebola viral haemorrhagic fever infection in Zaire in May. Three hundred and sixteen people were infected and 245 died - a 78% case-fatality rate. Ebola virus is transmitted by direct contact with blood secretions or body fluids from an infected person. There is no specific treatment; control depends on strict barrier nursing and infection control techniques for infected patients. The natural reservoir of the Ebola virus is not known. Appropriate agencies in the UK were alerted about the possibility of infection in anyone returning from the area, and how expected cases should be managed; no cases were reported outside the infected area in Zaire.

The spread of known pathogens also continued to cause concern. The diphtheria epidemic in the Russian Federation and the Ukraine continued and extended to other Newly Independent States of the former Soviet Union. There was also some evidence to indicate that tuberculosis, already resurgent in many developing countries, was increasing in several eastern European countries[1].

Reference

1. World Health Organization. Tuberculosis trends in Central and Eastern Europe. *Weekly Epidemiol Rec* 1995: **70:** 21-4.

(k)   Travel-related disease

In September, the UK Health Departments, in conjunction with the PHLS CDSC, published *Health information for overseas travel*[1], which draws together health information for doctors and other health professionals who advise travellers. It is intended as a companion volume to the Memorandum *Immunisation against infectious disease*[2], and replaces the travel section (but not the chapters on individual vaccines) in that book.

Malaria

A total of 2,055 cases of imported malaria were reported to the Malaria Reference Laboratory in 1995, compared with 1,887 in 1994 and 1,922 in 1993.

Of these, 1,113 (54%) were due to the potentially more serious *Plasmodium falciparum* malaria, compared with 1,176 (62%) in 1994 and 1,084 (56%) in 1993. Four patients died. As in previous years, more cases of *Plasmodium falciparum* malaria were acquired in West Africa than any other area, whereas most *Plasmodium vivax* malaria was acquired in Asia.

Hepatitis A

The PHLS received 1,689 laboratory reports of hepatitis A from England during 1995, of which 220 (13%) included a history of travel abroad. However, many reports do not record a travel history.

Typhoid

The PHLS received 265 reports of typhoid, 153 of paratyphoid A and 17 of paratyphoid B infections in 1995. Most were acquired in the Indian sub-continent.

Cholera

Forty three cases of cholera were notified during 1995, compared with 50 in 1994. The PHLS Laboratory of Enteric Pathogens confirmed and typed isolates from ten cases of cholera imported into England and Wales, all of which were *Vibrio cholerae* serogroup 01 biotype El Tor.

Legionnaires' disease

Eighty-six of the 159 cases of Legionnaires' disease reported in England and Wales during 1995 were defined as probably or possibly acquired abroad, compared with 77 of 158 cases in 1994. The European reporting system for travel-related cases of Legionnaires' disease, which is co-ordinated by the PHLS, continued to identify clusters related to a single destination which would have gone unrecognised without this collaboration. An outbreak associated with a hotel in Kusadasi, Turkey, highlighted the need for greater awareness of Legionnaires' disease and its control among operators in the travel industry. A joint seminar involving the Department, the PHLS and the travel industry was scheduled for Spring, 1996.

Other imported diseases

A variety of other imported infections were reported, including arboviruses, filaria, hookworm, leishmaniasis, schistosomiasis and strongyloides. Dengue is the commonest arbovirus reported; imported cases of dengue fever have increased in England and Wales since the late 1980s and reached 465, diagnosed serologically, in 1994[3]. An estimated 50 million cases of this infection occur world wide annually. The geographical distribution is similar to malaria, but dengue virus is primarily associated with urban rather than rural areas. Epidemics of both dengue and dengue haemorrhagic fevers were reported to be spreading through Central and South America during 1995, with at least 38 deaths.

References

1. Department of Health, Welsh Office, Scottish Office Home and Health Department, Northern Ireland Department of Health and Social Security, PHLS Communicable Disease Surveillance Centre. *Health information for overseas travel.* London: HMSO, 1995.
2. Department of Health. *Immunisation against infectious disease.* London: HMSO, 1992.
3. Communicable Disease Surveillance Centre. Dengue: current epidemics and risks to travellers. *Commun Dis Rep* 1995; **5**: 197.

CHAPTER 7

ENVIRONMENTAL HEALTH AND TOXICOLOGY

(a) Chemical and physical agents in the environment

(i) *Small Area Health Statistics Unit*

The Small Area Health Statistics Unit (SAHSU), based at the London School of Hygiene and Tropical Medicine, is funded by Government to investigate claims of unusual clusters of disease or ill-health in the vicinity of point sources of pollution from chemicals and/or radiation, such as industrial installations[1,2].

During 1995, the SAHSU published a study of cancer incidence and mortality near the Baglan Bay petrochemical works, field work for which was completed in 1994[2]; a general excess incidence of all cancer and of larynx cancer was observed, but was consistent with findings for the region and not thought to be related to emissions from the plant[3]. A number of other studies were completed but not published during the year. A study of cancer incidence near municipal solid waste incinerators was reassuring, although a small, probably artifactual, raised incidence of liver cancer will be investigated further. A study of angiosarcoma of the liver near vinyl chloride sites found no confirmed non-occupational cases. A study of leukaemia incidence near high-power radio transmitters found no more than a weak association.

In addition, the SAHSU continued to make a major contribution to the development of the methodology for investigating disease in small areas.

(ii) *Air pollution*

In late 1995, two reports from the Committee on the Medical Effects of Air Pollutants (COMEAP) were published[4,5]. The first, *Asthma and outdoor air pollution*[4], considered available evidence on the possible effects of non-biological air pollutants on both the initiation of asthma and the provocation of asthma attacks. The prevalence of asthma and other atopic diseases has increased dramatically during the past 30 years, but the Committee was not convinced that this worldwide problem is solely or even largely due to air pollution. Nevertheless, it was accepted that the provocation of asthma attacks and the worsening of symptoms in asthmatic patients may both be associated with raised levels of pollutants such as can occur in the United Kingdom (UK). In particular, data indicate that, although the effect is not large, admissions to hospital for treatment of acute exacerbations of asthma increase during air pollution episodes.

The second report, *Non-biological particles and health*[5], considered the rapidly accumulating evidence about possible effects on health both of short-term variations in concentrations of airborne particles and of raised long-term average levels of particles. The report concluded that the widely reported associations between daily concentrations of particles and effects on health reflect a real relation, and that although no clear mechanism to explain these effects has emerged, it would be imprudent not to regard the associations as causal. The Committee considered and recorded a number of attempts to quantify the health effects, but the lack of UK data made it impossible to verify the accuracy of predictions. The COMEAP also concluded that studies on the effects on health of raised long-term average particle concentrations were sound, though fewer than those for short-term variations, and advised that the reported associations should be regarded as causal.

These findings have been used by the Department of the Environment's (DoE's) Expert Panel on Air Quality Standards (EPAQS) to recommend an ambient air quality standard for particles. The recommendation refers to a measure known as PM10 (essentially the mass of particles of diameter less than 10 µm). The standard, 50 µg/m^3, is defined in terms of a 24-hour running average. The Panel accepted that, although exposure to 50 µg/m^3 would not be expected to harm the very large majority of individuals, effects may still be measurable at a population level. The annual average concentration in most urban areas is about 26 µg/m^3, and the Panel recommended this be reduced. In addition, the EPAQS recommended an air quality standard for sulphur dioxide of 100 parts per billion (ppb), measured as a running 15-minute average because of the rapid effects of sulphur dioxide on the respiratory system.

The Advisory Group on the Medical Aspects of Air Pollution Episodes published its final report *Health effects of exposures to mixtures of air pollutants*[6] in November. This completed a series of four reports which have helped to guide thinking on the effects of air pollutants on health. The Group concluded that additive effects could be expected when exposure to pollutant mixtures occurred, but that there was no evidence of any dramatic 'cocktail effect'.

The research initiative on air pollution and health[7] is now well under way, with 20 projects approved for funding by DH, DoE or the Medical Research Council (MRC). This new research programme will help to resolve some of the remaining questions about the effects of air pollutants on health.

(iii)   Committee on Medical Aspects of Radiation in the Environment

The Committee on Medical Aspects of Radiation in the Environment (COMARE) continued work on two reports in 1995. The first, a joint report with the Radioactive Waste Management Advisory Committee (RWMAC), published in May, was concerned with the potential health effects and possible sources of radioactive particles found in the vicinity of the Dounreay nuclear establishment[8]. This report contained important recommendations on environmental monitoring practices and considerations for the future of the intermediate-level waste shaft at Dounreay.

The second report[9], which will be published in Spring 1996, deals with the incidence of cancer and leukaemia in young people living in the village of Seascale near to the Sellafield nuclear site, and describes further studies since the publication of the report of the Black Advisory Group in 1984[10].

(iv)   Environment and health

DH continued to advise other Government Departments on health implications of chemicals in the environment in support of policy development and regulatory activity by those Departments. The MRC Institute for Environment and Health has carried out a number of projects on public health aspects of chemicals in the environment for DH and the DoE.

A major action agreed in the World Health Organization's (WHO's) environmental health action plan for Europe (EHAPE) was that each country would prepare its own national environmental health action plan (NEHAP) by 1997. The WHO invited the UK to be one of six countries to pilot the development of NEHAPs; these countries agreed to prepare their pilot plans by mid-1996 to test the feasibility of developing plans in the way envisaged in the EHAPE, and to serve as a guide for other countries to develop their own plans. The UK NEHAP will build on, and place more clearly into the public health context, environmental and sustainable development strategies which have been formulated in recent years. It was published, in draft form, in August and public comments were invited by the end of October. The document is being revised to take account of this consultation.

The European Environment and Health Committee (EEHC), chaired by the Chief Medical Officer, met twice during 1995. The EEHC is monitoring the production of the pilot NEHAPs and will also take account of wider, transboundary issues which affect all or groups of its members.

(v)   Surveillance of diseases possibly due to non-infectious environmental hazards

The monitoring of non-infectious diseases is less well developed than that for communicable diseases. There is a wide variety of chemicals in the environment and in most cases the links between such agents and possible health effects are not clearly established. Following recommendations of the Abrams Committee[11], an expert Working Group was set up and reported to the Chief Medical Officer in 1994[12]. During 1995, DH held discussions with colleagues from the NHS and other Government Departments about the nature of support needed by those responsible for the surveillance of non-infectious diseases which might be due to environmental factors, both with regard to the monitoring of ill-health possibly associated with relatively low levels of chemicals in the environment and to the related activity of response to chemical accidents.

Support may be needed to identify hazards to health from specific sites or substances; to assess likely exposures of individuals and the pathways involved;

and to assess risks arising from exposure to such hazards in the UK. It is clear that a number of organisations fulfil distinct, though interconnected, roles in this field. However, those delivering health services can have difficulty in finding the right source of advice quickly. Assessment of existing services, with a view to improving access to them and to identifying gaps in their provision, is under way.

References

1. Department of Health. *On the State of the Public Health: the annual report of the Chief Medical Officer of the Department of Health for the year 1991.* London: HMSO, 1992; 152.
2. Department of Health. *On the State of the Public Health: the annual report of the Chief Medical Officer of the Department of Health for the year 1994.* London: HMSO, 1995; 192.
3. Sans S, Elliott P, Kleinschmidt I et al. Cancer incidence and mortality near the Baglan Bay petrochemical works, South Wales. *Occup Environ Med* 1995; **52**: 217-24.
4. Department of Health, Committee on the Medical Effects of Air Pollutants. *Asthma and outdoor air pollution.* London: HMSO, 1995.
5. Department of Health, Committee on the Medical Effects of Air Pollutants. *Non-biological particles and health.* London: HMSO, 1995. Chair: Professor Stephen Holgate.
6. Department of Health, Advisory Group on the Medical Aspects of Air Pollution Episodes. *Health effects of exposures to mixtures of air pollutants: 4th report of the Advisory Group on the Medical Aspects of Air Pollution Episodes.* London: HMSO, 1995.
7. Department of Health. *On the State of the Public Health: the annual report of the Chief Medical Officer of the Department of Health for the year 1994.* London: HMSO, 1995; 192-4.
8. Committee on Medical Aspects of Radiation in the Environment, Radioactive Waste Management Advisory Committee. *Report on potential health effects and possible sources of radioactive particles found in the vicinity of the Dounreay nuclear establishment.* London: HMSO, 1995.
9. Committee on Medical Aspects of Radiation in the Environment. *Fourth report: the incidence of cancer and leukaemia in young people in the vicinity of the Sellafield site, West Cumbria; further studies and an update of the situation since the publication of the report of the Black Advisory Group in 1984.* London: Department of Health (in press).
10. Department of Health. *Investigation of the possible increased incidence of cancer in West Cumbria: report of the Independent Advisory Group.* London: HMSO, 1984. Chair: Sir Douglas Black.
11. Department of Health. *Public health responsibilities of the NHS and the roles of others.* London: Department of Health, 1993 (Miscellaneous Circular: MISC(93)56).
12. Department of Health. *On the State of the Public Health: the annual report of the Chief Medical Officer of the Department of Health for the year 1994.* London: HMSO, 1995; 195-6.

(b) Toxicological safety

(i) Food chemical hazards

The environmental contaminants dioxins have been discussed in previous Reports[1,2,3]. For most people, the greatest exposure to dioxins is from the diet and, in particular, from fatty foods and milk. During the year, the Committee on Toxicity of Chemicals in Food, Consumer Products and the Environment (COT) followed up its earlier assessment of dioxins[4] by reviewing a draft health assessment from the United States (US) Environmental Protection Agency (EPA)[5]. The EPA identified the same key targets for dioxins as had the COT - the immune system, reproduction and development, and cancer. The COT identified no new data in the EPA report which altered its previous hazard assessment of dioxins, and rejected the risk assessment model used by the EPA to derive a 'safe' level of exposure for human beings, based on animal carcinogenicity data, as insufficiently reliable for this purpose. The COT confirmed its tolerable daily intake (TDI) for dioxins of up to 10 picograms per kilogram bodyweight (pg/kg bw): current intakes of dioxins by the general population are around 1 pg/kg bw daily[6].

The COT also reviewed new toxicological studies on the artificial sweetener cyclamate, which has not been permitted for use in the UK since 1969. Cyclamate can be converted in the body to cyclohexylamine (CHA). Most people convert less than 0.1% of ingested cyclamate to CHA, but a small proportion of the population can convert up to 60%. CHA can damage the testes of laboratory rats when fed above a threshold level for 3 weeks or more. The new studies investigated the susceptibility of monkeys to this effect and showed that, in terms of plasma concentrations, monkey testes are as sensitive to CHA as those of rats. However, the severity of the effect was less and considered likely to be reversible. The COT regarded this and the information on a threshold in rats as reassuring, and set an acceptable daily intake (ADI) for cyclamate of up to 6 mg/kg bw. Cyclamate will again be permitted for use as a sweetener in the UK from 1 January 1996 following the introduction of harmonised legislation on sweeteners in all European Union (EU) Member States[7]. At the levels of use permitted in this legislation, it is not anticipated that the ADI will be exceeded.

Further information on topics reviewed by the COT and its sister Committees can be found in the Committees' annual report for 1995[8].

(ii)   Potential chemical carcinogens

Carbaryl is an insecticide used in pesticide products, medicines to control head lice and veterinary products. Following the submission of new carcinogenicity data in animals, the Advisory Committee on Pesticides (ACP) reviewed this compound with the advice of the Committee on Carcinogenicity of Chemicals in Food, Consumer Products and the Environment (COC), and the related Committee on Mutagenicity (COM). The COM concluded that there was no substantial evidence that carbaryl was a DNA-reactive mutagen in vivo, and the COC noted that since no other causal explanation could be provided for the increased incidence of vascular tumours in mice and bladder tumours in rats, it would be prudent to consider carbaryl as a potential carcinogen in human beings[9].

In the light of these recommendations, and of the absence of reports of tumours being associated with carbaryl use in human beings, the ACP recommended action to avoid unnecessary exposure by withdrawal of pesticides containing carbaryl from non-professional use and restriction of professional use to minimise operator exposure, and the Committee on Safety of Medicines recommended restriction of human medicinal use by reclassifying carbaryl preparations as prescription only medicines (see page 203).

(iii)   Traditional and herbal remedies

On 1 January, new medicines legislation[10] came into force. Herbal remedies which are sold or supplied in certain circumstances (as described in Section 12 of the Medicines Act 1968[11]) are not covered by the new regulations and continue to be exempt from licensing. Potent herbs continue to be restricted to supply on a prescription only basis[12], or through pharmacies or via herbal practitioners below a maximum dose[13]. Unlicensed herbal remedies may also be covered by the general provisions of the Food Safety Act 1990[14]. These controls provide an adequate basis to take action to secure public health.

Occasional instances of ill-effects potentially linked to traditional remedies have been reported[15,16,17,18,19]. The COT published recommendations[20] based on consideration of some of these cases. The number of cases is small (around 15 published in 1995), and evidence of a causal link and the responsible agent is not always clear, and the incidence of adverse reactions among people who take traditional remedies is unknown. Various initiatives to improve understanding of the risks are under discussion, and an investigation of the consumption of traditional remedies in patients with chronic diseases in a hospital serving many ethnic minority communities was commissioned.

(iv)   Novel foods

The safety of a wide range of novel foods was considered during the year by the Advisory Committee on Novel Foods and Processes (ACNFP), an independent expert committee that advises Government Ministers.

The Committee evaluated a particular strain of *Enterococcus faecium*, derived from intestinal flora isolates from people in part of the former USSR, for use as a novel starter culture in the production of cultured milk products (eg, yoghurt). The evaluation of this organism centred on its history and identification, as well as the specification and quality control criteria used to ensure a consistent product. Detailed consideration was given to data that indicated that this strain of *Enterococcus faecium* was generally sensitive to antibiotics and, in particular, that it did not contain any of the recognised genetic material encoding for resistance to the antibiotic vancomycin (vancomycin-resistant strains of *Enterococcus faecium* have been associated with clinical infections in some hospitals). The Committee also welcomed the decision of the company involved to deposit samples of their organism in recognised culture collections, for possible future reference purposes.

The ACNFP also completed its evaluation of the food safety of the seeds of the 'sweet' lupin, *Lupinus angustifolius*, a variety that contains lower levels of the alkaloids present in many other lupin varieties. Lupin seeds can be processed to produce food ingredients (flour or protein isolates) or can be used instead of soya beans in the production of oriental fermented food products. In common with many other proteinaceous food products, including legumes, there is some evidence to suggest that lupin-based foods may elicit allergenic reactions in

189

susceptible individuals. The ACNFP recommended that information on this possibility be made available to relevant health professionals, and also to allergy support groups[21].

The Committee has recommended food safety clearance for a number of genetically modified (GM) crop plants used to produce processed food products (maize modified to confer resistance to an insect pest, two oilseed rape varieties modified to confer resistance to particular herbicides and a tomato modified to improve processing characteristics)[21]. Clearance was also recommended for a GM tomato to be eaten fresh which has been modified to delay fruit softening, thereby allowing the tomatoes to ripen on the plant without compromising subsequent shelf-life. The development of some of these GM crop plants has involved the use of selective marker genes, including genes for resistance to antibiotics, which may still be present in the final transformed plant. From experience gained in these evaluations, the Committee will consider further its guidance on the criteria used to assess the acceptability of such marker genes in GM foods.

(v)   Pesticides

The UK has revised its system for the approval of pesticides to meet the requirements of new EC systems for authorisation of plant protection products or agricultural pesticides, established by EC Directive 91/414/EEC. The speed of evaluation required means that the UK's two-tiered system, whereby the Scientific Sub-committee on Pesticides (SCP) evaluates applications for pesticide approvals and makes a recommendation to the Advisory Committee on Pesticides (ACP), is no longer feasible. An Inter-Departmental Secretariat has therefore been established to meet as frequently as required to deal with approvals and reviews. The ACP will remain the principal source of independent scientific advice; the SCP will be disbanded in March 1996. The first meeting of the new Inter-Departmental Secretariat took place in December 1995.

Routine monitoring by the Working Party on Pesticide Residues (WPPR) of pesticide residues in carrots found that some individual roots had high concentration of certain organophosphorus insecticides used to control carrot fly. The ACP recommended that action be taken to reduce the residue levels. The ACP endorsed current food hygiene advice to wash thoroughly and prepare fruit and vegetables before use. The approvals of these pesticides on carrots was changed to limit the number of times they can be applied each year.

Samples of human fat for measurement of organochlorine residues were collected during the year; assays will be done in 1996, when collection is complete.

(vi)   Veterinary products

UK Health Departments are responsible, with the Ministry of Agriculture, Fisheries and Food (MAFF), for the authorisation of veterinary medicines. DH continued to provide advice to the MAFF on the human safety of veterinary drugs. DH officials attended meetings of the Veterinary Products Committee (VPC) and the VPC's Human Adverse Reactions Appraisal Panel. Expert Committees (COT, COM and COC) gave detailed advice on the toxicology of carbaryl (see page 188), oxibendazole and thiabendazole - all of which are used as veterinary medicinal products. Toxicological advice was given to the EC's Committee on Veterinary Medicinal Products on consumer safety aspects involved in the setting of statutory European maximum residue limits (MRLs) for veterinary drugs. DH provided toxicological and microbiological advice to the MAFF with regard to human safety aspects of applications for approval of animal feeds and feed additives.

DH is represented on the membership of the Advisory Group on Veterinary Residues, which met for the first time on 24 July. This Group deals with surveillance of food for residues resulting from the use of veterinary products.

In 1994, regulations[22] were brought in under the Medicines Act 1968[11] to ensure that those purchasing organophosphorus (OP) sheep dips had obtained a Certificate of Competence issued by the National Proficiency Tests Council. These regulations came fully into force in April 1995. DH, together with MAFF and the Health and Safety Executive (HSE), are jointly funding a study into the health of sheep dippers. This follows recommendations from the VPC, and its medical and scientific panel, for a carefully designed and targeted epidemiological study. A tender from the Institute of Occupational Medicine in Edinburgh, working in combination with the Institute of Neurological Sciences in Glasgow, was accepted and began in November. In October, a short article in *CMO's Update* reminded doctors of the possible acute and long-term effects of OP sheep dips[23].

References

1. Department of Health. *On the State of the Public Health: the annual report of the Chief Medical Officer of the Department of Health for the year 1988.* London: HMSO, 1989; 169-71.
2. Department of Health. *On the State of the Public Health: the annual report of the Chief Medical Officer of the Department of Health for the year 1991.* London: HMSO, 1992; 159-60.
3. Department of Health. *On the State of the Public Health: the annual report of the Chief Medical Officer of the Department of Health for the year 1992.* London: HMSO, 1993; 180-1.
4. Ministry of Agriculture, Fisheries and Food. *Dioxins in food: 31st report of the Steering Group on Chemical Aspects of Food Surveillance.* London: HMSO, 1992; 46-9 (Food Surveillance Paper no. 31).
5. United States Environmental Protection Agency. *Health assessment document for 2,3,7,8-tetrachlorodibenzo-p-dioxin (TCDD) and related compounds: external review draft.* Washington DC, USA: US Environmental Protection Agency, 1994 (Doc no. EPA/600/BP-92/001a).
6. Ministry of Agriculture, Fisheries and Food. *Dioxins in food.* London: Ministry of Agriculture, Fisheries and Food, 1995 (Food Safety Information Bulletin no. 63).
7. Commission of the European Community. European Parliament and Council Directive of 30 June 1994 on sweeteners for use in foodstuffs (EC/94/35). *Official J European Communities* no. L 237, 10 September 1994; 3-8.
8. Department of Health. *Annual report of the Committees on Toxicity, Mutagenicity, Carcinogenicity of Chemicals in Food, Consumer Products and the Environment: 1995.* London: HMSO (in press).
9. Department of Health. *Carbaryl.* London: Department of Health, 1995 (Professional Letter: PL/CMO(95)4, PL/CNO(95)3).

10. *The Medicines for Human Use (Marketing Authorisations etc.) Regulations 1994.* London: HMSO, 1994 (Statutory Instrument: SI 1994 no. 3144).
11. *The Medicines Act 1968.* London: HMSO, 1968.
12. *The Medicines (Products other than Veterinary Drugs) (Prescription Only) Order 1983.* London: HMSO, 1983 (Statutory Instrument: SI 1983 no. 1212).
13. *The Medicines (Retail Sale or Supply of Herbal Remedies) Order 1977.* London: HMSO, 1977 (Statutory Instrument: SI 1977 no. 2130).
14. *The Food Safety Act 1990.* London: HMSO, 1990.
15. Perharic L, Shaw D, Leon C, de Smet PA, Murray VS. Possible association of liver damage with the use of Chinese herbal medicine for skin disease. *Vet Hum Toxicol* 1995; **37**: 562-6.
16. Vautier G, Spiller R. Safety of complementary medicines should be monitored. *BMJ* 1995; **311**: 633.
17. Kane JA, Kane SP, Jain S. Hepatitis induced by traditional Chinese herbs; possible toxic components. *Gut* 1995; **36**: 146-7.
18. Shaw D, House I, Kolev S, Murray V. Should herbal medicines be licensed? *BMJ* 1995; **311**: 451-2.
19. Bayly GR, Braithwaite RA, Sheehan TM, Dyer NH, Grimley C, Ferner RE. Lead poisoning from Asian traditional remedies in the West Midlands: report of a series of five cases. *Hum Exper Toxicol* 1995; **14**: 24-8.
20. Department of Health. *Annual report of the Committees on Toxicity, Mutagenicity and Carcinogenicity of Chemicals in Food, Consumer Products and the Environment: 1994.* London: HMSO, 1995.
21. Department of Health, Ministry of Agriculture, Fisheries and Food. *Advisory Committee on Novel Foods and Processes: annual report: 1995.* London: Ministry of Agriculture, Fisheries and Food (in press).
22. *The Medicines (Veterinary Drugs) (Pharmacy and Merchants' List) (Amendment) Order 1994.* London: HMSO, 1994 (Statutory Instrument: SI 1994 no. 599).
23. Department of Health. Organophosphate sheep dips. *CMO's Update* 1995; **7**: 6.

CHAPTER 8

MEDICAL EDUCATION, TRAINING AND STAFFING

(a) Junior doctors' hours

The 1991 'New Deal'[1] introduced a timetable for the reduction of junior doctors' hours. By September 1995, just 295 - or 1% of all junior doctors - were in hard-pressed on-call posts contracted for more than 72 hours per week (compared with 1,676 on 31 December 1994); these few remaining posts are being tackled as a priority. Further action, including a review of working patterns, will also be necessary to reduce actual hours worked above the 56-hour limit and to cut work intensity - areas where progress has been slower.

The Department of Health (DH) continues to support the 'New Deal' with central funds. The cost in 1995/96 is £64 million, including an additional £14 million. This brings the total spent on the 'New Deal' since its launch to £180 million. Between 1991 and September 1995, this money has been used to fund an extra 1,252 senior doctor posts (including 1,052 consultants) expressly set up to help to reduce junior doctors' hours. Regions also developed many local projects, including extra nursing and support workers, and further improvements in living conditions.

Regional Task Forces are using a range of measures to reduce junior doctors' hours. 1995 has seen a wider take-up of new working patterns and the development of effective skill-mix initiatives across all hospital grades, notably the growth of nurse practitioner posts.

DH is now looking more closely at levels of work intensity within overall contracted hours, and at the end of the year agreed a revised system for increasing out-of-hours payments where work intensity remained too high. The Department has been working with the junior doctors themselves to ensure that actual hours of work are accurately monitored, and Regional Task Forces now involve junior doctors in the validation of these statistics. Despite considerable improvements, there remains a hard core of problem posts which need particular attention.

Reference

1. Department of Health. *Hours of work of doctors in training: the new deal.* London: Department of Health, 1991 (Executive Letter: EL(91)82).

(b) Advisory Group on Medical and Dental Education, Training and Staffing and the Specialist Workforce Advisory Group

The Advisory Group on Medical and Dental Education, Training and Staffing (AGMETS) was set up in late 1994 to advise Ministers and the National Health

Service (NHS) Executive on medical and dental education, training and staffing matters[1]. It is supported by a number of sub-groups and provides a single forum in which staffing policies can be considered in an integrated and co-ordinated manner, extending beyond hospital and community medical and dental staff to cover some general practice and public health issues.

The overall aim of medical staffing policy is to enable the NHS to secure an adequate supply of appropriately trained doctors. Within this overall aim, the AGMETS is developing new arrangements for medical staffing which will increase the involvement of the NHS locally, and improve the balance between central and local planning. The main features of these arrangements are:

— the close involvement of managers (Trusts and purchasers), the profession and the NHS Executive;

— a 'quality framework' to assist Trusts and purchasers to focus on medical staffing quality;

— greater emphasis on Trusts' medical staffing plans, which should conform to the 'quality framework' and have the support of main purchasers; *and*

— aggregation of Trusts' plans for workforce planning.

As part of this approach, local managers and Regional Offices will be able to take advice from local medical workforce advisory groups.

Specialist Workforce Advisory Group

The Specialist Workforce Advisory Group (SWAG) is established under the AGMETS umbrella, and also includes representatives of the medical profession, medical Royal Colleges and the NHS. Its task is to advise on the number of specialist registrars needed to fulfil the demand for candidates for consultant appointments.

During the year, the SWAG secretariat met with representatives of all medical specialties to assess the number of higher specialist trainees needed; the Group also used information from surveys of NHS Trusts. It concluded that there is a need for a substantial increase in the number of specialist registrars; the SWAG's recommendations will be considered by the NHS Executive Board and Ministers early in 1996.

The SWAG's approach will be refined to fit within the principles being developed by the AGMETS - in particular to provide a more accurate means to identify the demand for specialists in the light of service developments and technological advances. Changes will also be made to ensure greater participation by NHS management and to take into account effects on general practice and employers' plans for the non-medical workforce. During the year, work progressed to establish the regional postgraduate deans' database, which will also assist the planning process.

Reference

1. Department of Health. *On the State of the Public Health: the annual report of the Chief Medical Officer of the Department of Health for the year 1994*. London: HMSO, 1995; 203-4.

(c)   Medical Workforce Standing Advisory Committee

The Medical Workforce Standing Advisory Committee (MWSAC) published its second report in June[1]. (This Committee had been known as the Medical Manpower Standing Advisory Committee until 1 February, when its name changed to reflect equality of opportunity and established usage.) Its report recommended that more doctors need to be trained in the United Kingdom (UK) to meet likely future demand. Taking account of cost implications and the capacity of medical schools, the MWSAC recommended a gradual increase in medical school intake for five years from 1996, to arrive at a maximum annual target intake of 4,970 by the year 2000, with no change to the current overseas student quota of 7.5% of total intake. The Government accepted this recommendation, which is now being implemented.

The Committee also discussed key issues that affect medical workforce planning, including advances in medical technology; management and medical audit skills of doctors; and changes to the skill-mix between health care professionals.

Reference

1. Department of Health Medical Workforce Standing Advisory Committee. *Planning the medical workforce: second report*. London: Department of Health, 1995.

(d)   Postgraduate and specialist medical education

Implementation within the NHS of the reform of specialist medical training in response to the recommendations of the report of the Working Group on Specialist Medical Training (the Calman report)[1], is being co-ordinated by a steering group chaired by Professor John Temple, regional postgraduate dean for the West Midlands. Progress has been made possible through the co-operation of the Conference of medical Royal Colleges, the Committee of Postgraduate Medical Deans, NHS management and the AGMETS.

The European Specialist Medical Qualifications Order 1995[2] will come into force on 12 January 1996, following extensive consultation and detailed negotiations with the medical Royal Colleges and the General Medical Council (GMC) during 1995. A key component of the Order is the establishment of the Specialist Training Authority (STA) of the medical Royal Colleges as the Competent Authority for specialist medical training in the UK. The STA will be legally responsible for ensuring that postgraduate medical training in the UK complies with the requirements of the European Union's (EU's) Directive on Specialist Medical Training, which includes the awarding of a Certificate of Completion of Specialist Training (CCST) to doctors who have successfully completed a specialist medical training programme. The Order also establishes the GMC as the UK's Competent Authority responsible for the mutual recognition of qualifications under the requirements of the EU Directive, and requires the GMC to maintain and publish the new Specialist Register.

The main route of entry onto the Specialist Register for doctors training in the UK will be through the award of a CCST; sub-specialty interests may also be recorded on this Register. However, there are routes for entry to the Specialist Register for other doctors - such as those in academic or research medicine, and those with overseas training equivalent to CCST standards. There are also transitional provisions to enable existing NHS consultants and other fully trained specialists to be entered onto the Specialist Register. From 1 January 1997, a doctor must be on the Specialist Register before taking up a substantive or honorary NHS consultant post.

The report of the Working Party on the Unified Training Grade[3], which outlined the educational framework for the new specialist registrar grade, was widely distributed early in the year for consultation. Many detailed comments from medical practitioners, the medical Royal Colleges, NHS managers and professional organisations were taken into account before the launch of the new grade on 1 December in two vanguard specialties - general surgery and diagnostic radiology. Interim guidance on the operation of the grade was issued in November[4]. A further version will be produced ahead of the transition period in all other specialties, which will begin on 1 April 1996 (the grade commissioning date) and continue in a rolling programme over the subsequent 12 months.

Detailed negotiations with British Medical Association (BMA) representatives on pay and terms and conditions in the specialist registrar grade took place towards the end of the year; the proposed new pay arrangements have been submitted to the Doctors' and Dentists' Review Body for consideration.

Three further Working Groups were established to look at how implementation of the training reforms would affect the training of overseas doctors, doctors in academic and research medicine and doctors in general practice. Reports from these Groups were issued for consultation in May[5]. Preliminary work towards implementation of their recommendations was started, and will be taken forward under the auspices of the AGMETS.

Management of postgraduate medical and dental education

A number of changes to the management of postgraduate medical and dental education were made throughout 1995 in preparation for the health Region re-organisation from 1 April 1996.

Postgraduate deans

Postgraduate medical and dental education is currently managed on a regional basis by a postgraduate dean; responsibility for the management of training for general medical practice is devolved to the regional adviser in general practice, and for dental training to the dean of postgraduate dentistry. An infrastructure of assistants, tutors, course organisers and postgraduate centre staff provides support at regional and local levels.

In June, the Minister for Health announced[6] that, from April 1996, postgraduate medical deans would be jointly appointed by universities and Regional Offices to interdependent university and civil service contracts. Regional advisers would normally also work part-time in the Regional Offices, with contracts similar to those of the deans. The Personnel Directorate of the NHS Executive has worked on the detail of this proposal in consultation with regions, universities and the individuals concerned. It was accepted that issues such as the location and size of the dean's organisation and employment arrangements for the staff working there should be determined locally, taking account of local needs and circumstances and existing budgets. As a result, deans' offices will be variously based at universities, health authorities or NHS Trusts.

Junior doctors' contracts

After discussions with the medical profession and other parties, it was decided that, from 1 April 1996, junior doctors' contracts of employment would be held by Trusts; the postgraduate deans will be responsible for ensuring that educational needs are met. The necessary legal powers were taken to ensure that junior doctors on training rotations could be employed by Trusts whilst maintaining their continuity of service for employment purposes.

Funding arrangements

From 1 April 1996, funding for postgraduate medical and dental education will be raised by a charge on purchasers of health care, to be known as the Medical and Dental Education Levy (MADEL). These funds will be administered regionally by the postgraduate deans on behalf of the NHS Executive; mechanisms have been developed to monitor the effective use of these budgets. The aim is to provide postgraduate deans with a budget from April 1996 which should cover broadly the same items as their current budget. It would support 50% of the basic salaries of full-time doctors in training and 100% of the salaries of part-time trainees, and the costs of study leave, the training infrastructure, local training managers and regional postgraduate management. Some transfers of funds both into and out of the levy will occur for particular items.

Some MADEL funds will be used to support postgraduate dental training, educational development, the Standing Committee on Postgraduate Medical and Dental Education (SCOPME), medical and dental National Advice Centres and some activities of the medical Royal Colleges in relation to the maintenance of standards in postgraduate medical and dental education.

Regional postgraduate deans have been advised of their budgets for 1996/97, which total over £500 million.

References

1. Department of Health. *Hospital doctors: training for the future: the report of the Working Group on Specialist Medical Training.* London: Department of Health, 1993. Chair: Dr Kenneth Calman.
2. *The European Specialist Medical Qualifications Order 1995.* London: HMSO, 1995 (Statutory Instrument: SI 1995 no. 3208).
3. NHS Executive. *Unified training grade: report of the Working Party on the Unified Training Grade.* Leeds: Department of Health, 1994.
4. NHS Executive, Welsh Office, Northern Ireland Department of Health and Social Services, Scottish Home and Health Department. *A guide to specialist registrar training.* London: Department of Health, 1995.
5. Department of Health. *Hospital doctors: training for the future: the report of the Working Group on Specialist Medical Training: supplementary reports by the Working Groups Commissioned to Consider the Implications for General Medical Practice, Overseas Doctors and Academic and Research Medicine Arising from the Principal Report.* London: Department of Health, 1995.
6. Department of Health. *Future of junior doctors' contracts settled.* London: Department of Health, 1995 (Press Release 95/313).

(e)   Equal opportunities for doctors and the part-time consultants scheme

Flexible training

At the end of 1995, 595 senior registrars and 350 career registrars were working in flexible training schemes. As an interim measure in preparation for the launch of the specialist registrar grade, the waiting lists for flexible training staffing approvals were abolished, which enabled 160 trainee doctors to start flexible training as soon as arrangements could be finalised locally.

The yearly senior registrar flexible training competition was also abolished, but replaced by arrangements for receipt of applications for staffing approval throughout the year. This arrangement will end, on a specialty by specialty basis, when each reaches its commissioning date for transition to the new specialist registrar grade.

Guidance for flexible trainees in the new specialist registrar grade has been included in guidance for the grade as a whole[1]. These arrangements were developed in 1995 from the consensus of comments received during consultation on the framework for the grade and discussions with the medical profession, including the postgraduate deans' Flexible Working Group and the Women in Surgical Training (WIST) scheme.

Part-time consultants scheme

There are currently 122 consultants working under the part-time consultants scheme. The first tranche of the scheme should be evaluated by July 1996. A decision on whether to extend the scheme will then be made.

Opportunity 2000

The third goal of Opportunity 2000[2] was to increase the percentage of women consultants from 15.5% in 1991 to 20% by 1994. Figures for September 1994 indicated that women consultants had increased to approximately 18% of the total consultant workforce. A new target has been set for 22% of consultant posts to be held by women by September 1998.

References

1. NHS Executive, Welsh Office, Northern Ireland Department of Health and Social Services, Scottish Office Home and Health Department. *A guide to specialist registrar training.* London: Department of Health, 1995.
2. NHS Executive. *Women in the NHS: an implementation guide to Opportunity 2000.* London: Department of Health, 1992.

(f)   Undergraduate medical and dental education

Steering Group on Undergraduate Medical and Dental Education and Research

Close co-operation between the NHS and universities is essential for the successful management of medical and dental education and research. The Steering Group on Undergraduate Medical and Dental Education and Research (SGUMDER) advises the Secretaries of State for Health and for Education and Employment on the arrangements for and service implications of undergraduate medical and dental education and research. Its membership includes senior representatives from the NHS and universities.

The SGUMDER's most important work has involved the development of robust joint working arrangements between universities and the NHS, known as the 'ten key principles'. The Group will shortly publish its fourth report, which includes a revision of these principles and makes recommendations for effective NHS/university liaison following the Health Authorities Act 1995[1].

Service Increment for Teaching

The Service Increment for Teaching and Research (SIFTR) funds the costs to the NHS of supporting the clinical teaching of medical undergraduates. In 1995/96, the SIFTR will be £541 million inclusive of capital charges, of which medical SIFT accounted for £367 million.

An Advisory Group was established in December 1994 to review the methodology and distribution of SIFT. The Group's report *SIFT into the future*[2] was published in May 1995[3], together with a consultation paper setting out proposals for changes to dental SIFT. The new arrangements for SIFT were announced by Ministers in October. The main objectives are:

— flexibility;

— improved accountability; *and*

— the creation of a stable framework within which changes can evolve.

The new arrangements for SIFT will take effect from 1 April 1996. New arrangements for dental SIFT will also come into effect on 1 April 1996, when Sheffield Health Authority will manage the national dental SIFT budget.

Undergraduate Medical Curriculum Implementation Support Scheme

In 1993, DH launched the Undergraduate Medical Curriculum Implementation Support Scheme to enable medical schools to appoint facilitators to help them to implement the curriculum changes outlined in the GMC's report *Tomorrow's doctors*[4]; a similar scheme exists for dental schools. Over £1.2 million were allocated for this purpose in 1995/96.

References

1. *Health Authorities Act 1995*. London: HMSO, 1995.
2. NHS Executive. *SIFT into the future: future arrangements for allocating funds and contracting for NHS service support and facilities for teaching undergraduate medical students: report of the Advisory Group on SIFT*. Leeds: Department of Health, 1995.
3. NHS Executive. *Undergraduate medical and dental education*. Wetherby (West Yorkshire): Department of Health, 1995 (Executive Letter: EL(95)63).
4. General Medical Council. *Tomorrow's doctors: recommendations on undergraduate medical education*. London: General Medical Council, 1993.

(g)   Medical (Professional Performance) Act

The Department has worked closely with the GMC to provide the legislative framework for proposed changes to procedures related to standards of professional performance. The Medical (Professional Performance) Act 1995[1] was enacted in November. The GMC is now developing its detailed procedures and committee rules with a view to the Act coming into force in 1997.

The Act also includes provisions to strengthen the GMC's powers to safeguard the public pending the full hearing of a case by allowing it to make interim suspension orders for six months instead of the present two months, and to allow these orders to be extended. The health committee of the GMC will also be able to impose suspension indefinitely when a doctor has already been suspended for two years, which will release sick doctors from the requirement to attend a hearing each year. These provisions will come into force on 1 May 1996.

Reference

1. *The Medical (Professional Performance) Act 1995*. London: HMSO, 1995.

(h)   Maintaining medical excellence

The report *Maintaining medical excellence*[1], which was published for consultation in August after a thorough review of existing guidance in relation to the identification of poor performance of doctors, emphasises the need for assuring and improving the quality and delivery of health care. The report makes a number of recommendations for improvements in the standard of professional performance to ensure that patients, in the NHS and the private sector alike, are treated by doctors whose professional skills and competence are of a satisfactory and safe standard. The need to identify and promote a network of support for doctors who, for various reasons, may not be performing as well as they should lies at the heart of the report. The review group emphasised the need to ensure that poor performance is identified at an early stage, and that appropriate remedial action is taken before serious problems occur.

A key recommendation was the introduction of systems for mentoring for all hospital medical staff. Mentoring is intended to offer doctors professional contact and support from a respected colleague in their own professional field, and to provide them with the opportunity to review issues of professional practice and development.

The report also stresses the importance of identifying any difficulties which may arise during undergraduate training, the need to improve methods of supervising pre-registration house officer posts, and calls for fuller assessment of the suitability of doctors for vocational training. It also discusses other means of helping to improve performance and to reduce the risk of problems developing later on in a professional career. Doctors must also be actively encouraged to take advantage of continuing medical education (CME) to improve their existing skills, to develop new skills and to keep themselves up-to-date with current medical thinking and practices. The medical Royal Colleges have been developing their approaches to CME, and this work is welcomed.

Maintaining medical excellence[1] highlights the need for new and revised guidance to help Health Authorities and Trusts to identify the correct procedures to deal with individual cases of poor performance. A great deal of the guidance currently in use pre-dates the recent reforms that have taken place in the NHS, and DH is working closely with employers and the BMA to consider recommendations for new procedures.

Maintaining medical excellence[1] is an important part of the work the Department is taking forward to ensure and improve the quality of medical practice and performance. The challenge for the medical profession is to provide programmes which meet the needs of the NHS as a whole as well as individual doctors.

Reference

1. Department of Health. *Maintaining medical excellence: review of guidance on doctors' performance: final report.* London: Department of Health, 1995.

(i)   Locum doctors

The report of the Locums Working Group on hospital locum doctors was published for consultation in January[1].   The report contained recommendations to reduce the dependence of hospitals on locum doctors and to improve quality control procedures.   Various measures for both short-term and long-term action were recommended, and a draft code of practice in locum appointments was proposed.   The results of this consultation process and the possible links with other measures related to professional performance, staffing, and continuing medical education are under consideration by the Department.

Reference

1. NHS Executive. *Hospital locum doctors: the report of the Locums Working Group: a consultative document.* Leeds: Department of Health, 1995.

CHAPTER 9

OTHER TOPICS OF INTEREST IN 1995

(a)   Medicines Control Agency

(i)   *Role and performance*

The Medicines Control Agency (MCA) is an executive agency which reports through its Chief Executive, Dr Keith Jones, to the Secretary of State for Health. Its role is to advise Ministers and to protect public health through the control of human medicines, and its primary concern is that medicines available to the public should meet the most stringent criteria for safety, efficacy and quality.

On behalf of Health Ministers (the Licensing Authority), the MCA approves medicines for marketing through the provision of a licence or marketing authorisation, monitors medicines after licensing, takes action to resolve drug safety concerns, licenses manufacturers and wholesale dealers, and carries out inspection and enforcement under the provisions of the Medicines Act 1968[1], associated United Kingdom (UK) legislation and relevant European Union (EU) Directives. The MCA also supports the work of the British Pharmacopoeia Commission in setting quality standards for drug substances. The MCA is financed by fees charged to the pharmaceutical industry, but aims to set these no higher than necessary and continuously reviews the quality of its service. It is responsible for medicines control policy within the Department of Health (DH) and represents the UK in pharmaceutical regulation within European and other international settings.

During 1995, the MCA met almost all of its key licensing and safety targets. The Agency continued to play a leading role in the new European Licensing Systems, acting as rapporteur for many of the products receiving centralised marketing authorisation. The volume of work brought to the Agency by the pharmaceutical companies was at record levels.

(ii)   *Legal reclassification of medicinal products*

The Prescription Only Medicine (POM) Order[2] was amended twice in 1995[3,4]. Two substances previously available for pharmacy sale (P) were reclassified as POMs for safety reasons. Carbaryl was reclassified because its potential carcinogenicity in animals led to concern that use without medical supervision might be hazardous to human beings (see page 190). Pancreatin formulations with a high lipase content were similarly reclassified because of a dose-related association with the development of ileo-caecal and large-bowel strictures. Five drug substances were reclassified to allow over-the-counter sale from pharmacies: fluconazole for vaginal candidiasis, hydroxyzine hydrochloride for pruritus, pyrantel embonate for enterobiasis, budesonide for seasonal allergic rhinitis and ketoconazole for seborrhoeic dermatitis. The existing exemption from POM classification for beclomethasone dipropionate was widened to include prophylaxis of hayfever. The maximum daily dose of pseudoephedrine available for pharmacy sale was increased, and three topical products which contain hydrocortisone were also reclassified as P.

New procedures for amending the legal classification of medicines from pharmacy sale to general sale list (GSL) were agreed, including regular amendment of the GSL Order[5] with prior consultation. In future, temporary GSL status will be granted only in exceptional circumstances. The GSL Order was amended[6] to include small packs of topical clotrimazole for athlete's foot and ibuprofen at limited dosage; the maximum dose of folic acid available on the GSL was raised to 500 micrograms to permit wider availability for the prophylaxis of neural tube defects to women planning a pregnancy (see page 147).

(iii)   Oral contraceptives

The Agency investigated the cardiovascular risks associated with combined oral contraceptives (OCs) as new evidence from epidemiological studies emerged between July and October 1995. A special meeting of the Committee on Safety of Medicines (CSM) was convened in October where the findings of three studies were considered. These showed a consistently increased risk of venous thromboembolism associated with OCs that contained desogestrel or gestodene, compared with those that contained levonorgestrel, which could not be accounted for by chance, bias or confounding. In view of the public health implications of these findings, the CSM recommended that OCs containing desogestrel or gestodene should only be used by women who are intolerant of other combined OCs and prepared to accept an increased risk of thromboembolism. The Committee advised that there was an urgent need to communicate the new advice with appropriate recommendations to the professions and the public. On 18 October, the chairman of the CSM wrote to all doctors to inform them of the new advice[7], and further information was distributed by the Chief Medical Officer in November[8].

(iv)   Pharmaceutical developments in the European Union

The new European Union (EU) marketing authorisation (licensing) system began operation on 1 January. Its new centralised and decentralised procedures, supported by the European Medicines Evaluation Agency (EMEA), are outlined below. The MCA played a leading role in the new procedures: it was rapporteur or co-rapporteur for 14 of the first 18 applications that were considered in the centralised procedure, conducted six of the first 16 inspections required of overseas manufacturers, and UK authorisations were the basis of more than 40% of mutual recognition applications in the decentralised procedure.

The MCA negotiated Commission Regulations governing variations to marketing authorisations and adverse reaction reporting. These were adopted in March, and completed the legislative base for the new EU authorisation system. The MCA also played an active part in the development of EU operational guidelines.

References

1. *The Medicines Act 1968*. London: HMSO, 1968.
2. *The Medicines (Products Other Than Veterinary Drugs) (Prescription Only) Order 1983*. London: HMSO, 1983 (Statutory Instrument: SI 1983 no. 1212).
3. *The Medicines (Products Other Than Veterinary Drugs) (Prescription Only) Amendment Order 1995*. London: HMSO, 1995 (Statutory Instrument: SI 1995 no. 1384).
4. *The Medicines (Products Other Than Veterinary Drugs) (Prescription Only) Amendment Order (Number 2) 1995*. London: HMSO, 1995 (Statutory Instrument: SI 1995 no. 3174).
5. *The Medicines (Products Other than Veterinary Drugs) (General Sale List) Order 1984*. London: HMSO, 1984 (Statutory Instrument: SI 1984 no. 769).
6. *The Medicines (Products Other Than Veterinary Drugs) (General Sale List) Amendment Order 1995*. London: HMSO, 1995 (Statutory Instrument: SI 1995 no. 3216).
7. Committee on Safety of Medicines. *Combined oral contraceptives and thromboembolism*. London: Committee on Safety of Medicines, 1995.
8. Department of Health. Venous thromboembolism and oral contraceptives that contain desogestrel or gestodene. *CMO's Update* 1995; **8**: 2.

(b)   European Medicines Evaluation Agency

The EMEA, based in London's Docklands, was established to support the new EU marketing authorisation (licensing) procedures which were set in place by a Council Regulation and three Directives adopted in 1993. The system began operation on 1 January 1995, although transitional arrangements apply until 1998. The legislation will provide a single EU pharmaceuticals authorisation system from 1998 with two components - centralised and decentralised. The centralised procedure will be mandatory for authorisations of biotechnology products and optional for authorisations of certain high-technology medicines; the decentralised procedure for other medicines is based on the principle of mutual recognition of Member States' authorisations, with binding arbitration in the event of disputes. This legislation was supplemented by a Council Regulation governing fees payable to the EMEA, which came into force in February.

The EMEA acts as a secretariat, providing administrative support to the centralised procedure by co-ordination of the existing scientific resources of Member States. In particular, it supports two committees of scientific experts nominated by the Member States to provide scientific advice to the European Commission on authorisation issues - the Committees on Proprietary Medicinal Products (CPMP) and Veterinary Medicinal Products (CVMP).

Establishment of the EMEA will enable rapid access to the whole EU pharmaceutical market by streamlining the authorisation of medicinal products, and its location in London is a key component of 'Prescribe UK' - the inward investment initiative launched to attract international pharmaceutical companies, particularly from the United States of America and Japan, to invest in the UK.

(c)   Medical Devices Agency

Role

The Medical Devices Agency (MDA) is an Executive Agency of the Department which reports through its Chief Executive, Mr Alan Kent, to the Secretary of

State for Health. The role of the Agency is to advise Ministers and safeguard public health by ensuring that all medical devices meet appropriate standards of safety, quality and performance, and comply with the relevant Medical Devices Directives of the European Union.

Developments in the European Union

The UK has played an active part in the initiatives and negotiations to bring about a single European market in medical devices.

The Active Implantable Medical Devices Regulations[1] came fully into force on 1 January 1995. All active implantable medical devices subsequently on sale must carry a CE marking, although there have been occasional exceptions to this requirement during 1995, where the Secretary of State for Health has allowed active implantable devices without such a marking to be used on humanitarian grounds.

The Medical Devices Regulations 1994[2] took effect on 1 January 1995, with a transition period until 13 June 1998. The Regulations introduced statutory control for the first time to a wide variety of products ranging from dressings to orthopaedic implants and computed tomography (CT) scanners.

Negotiation of the third Directive covering in-vitro diagnostic medical devices begins early in 1996. The Agency has convened a working group, which includes representatives of relevant professional associations, to advise on the UK's stance in these discussions.

The MDA acts as the UK's Competent Authority to implement the provisions of, and monitor compliance with, the EU Devices Directives, and to take any necessary enforcement action. The work of the Agency as a regulatory authority increased considerably during 1995. Eight independent certification organisations or Notified Bodies, which assess manufacturers' compliance against the essential requirements of the Regulations, were designated; and a programme of regular audit was instigated to assess the Notified Bodies' continued competence to carry out their functions satisfactorily. Additionally, 100 applications were received for clinical investigation approval. A panel of external assessors set up to assist the Competent Authority in assessing clinical investigation submissions, which comprises experts in both clinical and technical aspects of devices, has proved invaluable.

In October, the Medical Devices Fees Regulations[3], whereby the Agency now charges fees for Notified Body designation and clinical investigation assessment, were introduced.

Adverse incident reporting centre/vigilance system

During 1995, the MDA received over 4,100 reports of device-related adverse incidents, and investigated about 1,000 of these in depth. Approximately 2,000 less serious incidents were allocated for investigation by the manufacturer, with appropriate monitoring of progress and quality of response by the Agency.

With the introduction of the Medical Devices Directives, however, manufacturers are statutorily required to report all serious incidents related to CE-marked devices to the Competent Authority. Forty-nine such reports were received in 1995.

As a result of adverse incident investigations, six Hazard Notices, 33 Safety Notices and six Pacemaker Technical Notes were issued.

Evaluation programme

During the year, 135 reports were published; these evaluated a wide range of devices, include pathology test kits and radiological, dialysis and disability equipment.

Other publications

In 1995, a new series of publications called Device Bulletins were issued by the MDA: these contain guidance and information on more general device-related issues that arise from adverse incident investigations or repeated inquiries from health service users. Topics have included infusion systems[4] and the re-use of devices marked for single use only[5]. Additionally, after setting up a working group, the MDA published a report on alarms on monitoring devices[6], in response to Recommendation 11 of the Clothier Inquiry[7]. During 1995, the MDA also published guidance on the equipment and organisation involved in the transport of neonates[8] and produced a videotape of the previously published booklet *Doing no harm*[9], to introduce the Agency and its function to all health care professionals.

References

1. *The Active Implantable Medical Devices Regulations 1992*. London: HMSO, 1992 (Statutory Instrument: SI 1992 no. 3146).
2. *Medical Devices Regulations 1994*. London: HMSO, 1994 (Statutory Instrument: SI 1994 no. 3017).
3. *Medical Devices Fees Regulations*. London: HMSO, 1995 (Statutory Instrument: SI 1994 no. 2487).
4. Medical Devices Agency. *Infusion systems*. London: Department of Health, 1995 (Device Bulletin 9503).
5. Medical Devices Agency. *Re-use of medical devices supplied for single use only*. London: Department of Health, 1995 (Device Bulletin 9501).
6. Medical Devices Agency. *The report of the Expert Working Group on Alarms on Clinical Monitors in response to recommendation 11 of the Clothier Report: the Allitt Inquiry*. London: Medical Devices Agency, 1995.
7. Clothier C. *The Allitt Inquiry: independent inquiry relating to deaths and injuries on the children's ward at Grantham and Kesteven General Hospital during the period February to April 1991*. London: HMSO, 1994. Chair: Sir Cecil Clothier.
8. Medical Devices Agency. *Transport of neonates in ambulances*. London: Department of Health, 1995.
9. Medical Devices Agency. *Doing no harm*. London: Department of Health, 1994.

(d)   National Blood Authority

The National Blood Authority (NBA) was set up in April 1993, when it took over the management of the Bio-Products Laboratory and the International Blood Group Reference Laboratory. It also took over responsibility for the management of the former Regional Blood Transfusion Centres from Regional Health Authorities in April 1994.

During 1994, the NBA published proposals to reorganise the blood service on a national basis, so that it could effectively meet current and projected needs for blood and blood products. An independent panel was appointed to check that responses to the consultation document had been fully considered, and meetings were held with clinicians to ensure that their interests were properly reflected. In November 1995, Ministers announced that they had accepted the NBA proposals, which had been revised in the light of the consultation process.

The NBA will implement the proposed changes over a period of three to four years. Blood processing and testing will be consolidated at 10 of the existing 15 centres. However, all 15 centres will retain their blood banks, and two new blood banks will be added. The changes should enable emergency delivery of blood to all NHS hospitals to be guaranteed within two hours, for the first time. DH is setting up an independent national user group, chaired by Professor Edward Gordon-Smith, Professor of Haematology at St George's Hospital, London, to monitor the service provided to hospitals; the group's report will be published annually.

The NBA also plans to improve blood collection arrangements. It has introduced a new blood donor's charter[1], to be reviewed after a year, setting out what donors can expect from the blood service. Administration arrangements within the blood service are also to be concentrated at three zonal centres in London, Leeds and Bristol.

The goal of this reorganisation is to improve the safety, reliability and efficiency of the service and to meet the changing needs of the NHS. When the changes are fully implemented, savings should become available for improved patient care elsewhere in the health service.

Reference

1. Department of Health. *The patient's charter: blood donors: interim charter.* London: Department of Health, 1995.

(e)   National Biological Standards Board

The National Biological Standards Board (NBSB) is a non-Departmental public body set up in 1976 with a statutory duty[1,2] to assure the quality of biological substances used in medicine. The Board fulfils this function through its management of the National Institute for Biological Standards and Control (NIBSC). The NIBSC is a multidisciplinary scientific organisation which tests the quality, reliability and safety of biological medicines such as vaccines and products derived from human blood; develops the biological standards necessary for this testing; and conducts associated research.

The Board and the Institute work within the Government's overall public health programme to:

— respond to and advise on public health problems involving biological agents;

— address new developments in science and medicine; *and*

— take a leading role in developing the scientific basis for the control and standardisation of biological agents in Europe.

The NIBSC examines almost 2,000 batches of biological medicines annually, in addition to testing over 2,000 pools of plasma for virological safety. The Institute is designated an Official Medicines Control Laboratory within the EU and is one of only two such laboratories to have achieved independent quality accreditation for testing biological agents. This accreditation is to the internationally recognised quality standard EN45001.

The Institute is a World Health Organization (WHO) International Laboratory for Biological Standards and prepares and distributes the bulk of the world's international standards and reference materials. These activities are certified to the quality standard ISO9001.

References

1. *The Biological Standards Act 1975.* London: HMSO, 1975.
2. *The National Biological Standards Board (Functions) Order 1976.* London: HMSO, 1976 (Statutory Instrument: SI 1976 no. 917).

(f)   National Radiological Protection Board

The National Radiological Protection Board (NRPB) is a non-Departmental Public Body which reports to the Secretary of State for Health. The functions given to the Board[1,2] are:

— by means of research and otherwise, to advance the acquisition of knowledge about the protection of mankind from radiation hazards (for both ionising and non-ionising radiation; *and*

— to provide information and advice to persons (including Government Departments).

The NRPB's contribution to DH's Health of the Nation campaign is by a combination of formal advice, the publication of advisory reports and the provision of advice directly to health professionals and others involved with radiation work, as well as to the general public. Training courses are also run at the NRPB and within, or in conjunction with, academic or public health institutions. New training courses have been set up to cover health protection from lasers, ultraviolet radiation (UVR) and electromagnetic fields, and new medical courses for occupational physicians have been given. Radiation protection advisory visits and dosimetry services are provided to users of radiation equipment such as dental practitioners, hospitals and clinics, and industrial radiographers.

Formal Board advice was given during the year on the effects of UVR on human health. This statement[3] and the report of the Advisory Group on Non-ionising Radiation[4] received widespread publicity, which should have helped to raise the public's knowledge of the harmful effects of excess exposure to UVR. The Board has forged a medical link with the Dermatology Department at Oxford University to build up its clinical experience of skin cancers. The risks associated with exposures to electromagnetic fields remain a topical issue and the Advisory Group on Non-ionising Radiation continues to review the subject. The Board published a full re-assessment of the radiological impact of Seascale for the Committee on the Medical Aspects of Radiation in the Environment (COMARE)[5]. Additionally, a report was published on the risk of radiation-induced cancer at low doses and low dose-rates[6].

The WHO have approached the NRPB to become a Collaborating Centre for ionising and non-ionising radiation protection and negotiations have commenced. Support was given to the WHO for a conference on Chernobyl, held in November, and in writing the epidemiological part of its report for the international programme into the health effects of the Chernobyl accident.

The Board's *At-a-glance* leaflets remain very popular and cover fields such as medical radiation, radon and non-ionising radiation. Over one million of these leaflets have been produced and distributed, many to the public.

To achieve central cost savings, agreements were made during 1995 for the NRPB to assume the administrative support for the Administration of Radioactive Substances Advisory Committee (ARSAC) and the secretariat support for the COMARE. These changes will be implemented in 1996.

References

1. *The Radiological Protection Act 1970.* London: HMSO, 1970.
2. *Extensions of Functions Order 1974.* London: HMSO, 1974.
3. National Radiological Protection Board. *Board statement on effects of ultraviolet radiation on human health.* Oxford: National Radiological Protection Board, 1995 (Doc. NRPB 6, no. 2).
4. National Radiological Protection Board. *Health effects from ultraviolet radiation: report of an Advisory Group on Non-ionising Radiation.* Oxford: National Radiological Protection Board, 1995 (Doc. NRPB 6, no. 2).
5. Simmonds JR. *Risks of leukaemia and other cancers in Seascale from all sources of ionising radiation exposure.* Oxford: National Radiological Protection Board, 1995 (NRPB-R276).
6. National Radiological Protection Board. *Risk of radiation-induced cancer at low doses and low dose-rates for radiation protection purposes.* Oxford: National Radiological Protection Board, 1995 (Doc. NRPB 6, no. 1).

(g)   United Kingdom Transplant Support Service Authority

The UK Transplant Support Service Authority (UKTSSA) was established as a Special Health Authority on 1 April 1991 to provide a 24-hour support service to all transplant units in the UK and the Republic of Ireland, taking over the work of the UK Transplant Service. Its main functions include the matching and allocation of organs for transplantation on an equitable basis and in accordance with agreed methodologies; the provision of support and quality assurance to local tissue-typing laboratories; the maintenance and analysis of the national database of transplant information; and the production of audit reports on the status of transplantation and organ donation and use. The UKTSSA also provides a forum at which transplant and organ donation issues can be discussed and is responsible for the maintenance of the National Health Service (NHS) organ donor register, which was established in 1994. By December 1995, over 2.25 million people had registered their willingness to donate their organs in the event of sudden death.

(h)   Public Health Laboratory Service Board

The purpose of the Public Health Laboratory Service (PHLS) is to protect the population from infection, working collaboratively with other public health bodies both nationally and internationally. The Service was established in 1946, and the PHLS Board was formally constituted as a non-Departmental public body in 1960 to exercise functions which are embodied in statute in the National Health Service Act 1977[1], as amended by the Public Health Laboratory Service Act 1979[2]. The Board is accountable to the Secretary of State for Health and the Secretary of State for Wales.

The PHLS delivered services in 1995 through a network of 53 public health laboratories, distributed across England and Wales, providing clinical diagnostic microbiology services to 900 NHS customers, as well as food and environmental microbiology services for public health customers including over 400 local authorities. Over 10 million samples were processed, and the laboratories also assisted in the investigation of approximately 700 outbreaks of communicable disease during the year.

At the hub of this network are the Central Public Health Laboratory (CPHL) and the Communicable Disease Surveillance Centre (CDSC), which are located with the headquarters of the Service at Colindale. In 1995, the CPHL continued to develop its role as Britain's major reference centre for medical microbiology, in particular through the establishment of a new reference laboratory for *Campylobacter* infections. The main role of the CDSC is the national surveillance of infections and communicable diseases. During the year, the CDSC reviewed its protocols for surveillance of specific infections with a view to enhancing their effectiveness and improving prevention; issued guidance on the reporting of laboratory-confirmed infections[3]; and was at the forefront of European initiatives in communicable disease surveillance.

During 1995, the PHLS Board started to implement a new strategy based on the conclusions of a strategic review of the Service carried out in 1994[4]. This strategy entails the commitment of resources to a programme of service developments, including the strengthening of surveillance systems for hospital-acquired infections, improving the understanding of environmentally derived infections, increasing the application of molecular technology to microbiological investigations, and strengthening the training and education of public health professionals in the field of communicable diseases.

The service development strategy will be underpinned by a major re-organisation of the PHLS network of laboratories into 10 groups to enhance both their management and the effectiveness of the services that they provide. Two groups were formally established in April 1995; the remaining eight prepared detailed plans as the basis for their full establishment during 1996. This new management structure, together with further integration of the two national centres, will enable a greater focus on public health requirements and will further improve services to all users.

References

1. *The National Health Service Act 1977.* London: HMSO, 1977.
2. *The Public Health Laboratory Service Act 1979.* London: HMSO, 1979.
3. Public Health Laboratory Service. *Reporting to PHLS Communicable Disease Surveillance Centre: a guide for laboratories.* London: Public Health Laboratory Service, 1995.
4. Public Health Laboratory Service. *Report of a Strategic Review of the Public Health Laboratory Service.* London: Public Health Laboratory Service, 1994.

(i)   Microbiological Research Authority

The Centre for Applied Microbiology and Research (CAMR) at Porton Down was established as a Special Health Authority in April 1994 under the Board of the Microbiological Research Authority. In 1995, a research steering group was set up to provide systematic assessment of the research work commissioned and funded by DH. Membership of this group comprises representatives from the PHLS and DH, and two independent external assessors. Projects are grouped into the areas of pathogenesis, diagnostics, therapeutics, vaccines or environmental microbiology; they are assessed individually - for example, in terms of their scientific quality, relevance to policy, achievement towards project targets and value for money. Included in the current public health research programme are projects related to HIV, *Campylobacter*, verocytotoxin-producing *Escherichia coli* (VTEC) and *Salmonella*. An important area is vaccine development, and work is continuing at CAMR to develop vaccines against, for example, *Neisseria meningitidis*.

(j)   National Creutzfeldt-Jakob Disease Surveillance Unit

The National Creutzfeldt-Jakob Disease (CJD) Surveillance Unit continued to monitor the pattern of CJD in the UK. This Unit was set up in 1990 to monitor changes in the pattern of CJD in the UK. It investigates the incidence and

Table 9.1: *Creutzfeldt-Jakob disease (CJD) and Gerstmann-Straussler-Scheinker syndrome (GSS), United Kingdom, 1985-95*

Year	Creutzfeldt-Jakob disease			GSS	Total	Sporadic incidence/ million population*
	Sporadic	Iatrogenic	Familial			
1985	26	1	1	0	28	0.45
1986	26	0	0	0	26	0.45
1987	23	0	0	1	24	0.40
1988	21	1	1	0	23	0.36
1989	28	1	1	0	30	0.48
1990	26	5	0	0	31	0.45
1991	32	1	3	0	36	0.55
1992	44	2	4	1	51	0.76
1993	37	4	2	2	45	0.64
1994	53	1	2	3	59	0.92
1995†	36‡	4	1	2	43	0.62

* Based on UK population of 57.78 million (1991 Census update).
† Provisional figures.
‡ Includes 3 cases with unusual clinicopathological findings (new variant CJD [NVCJD]).
Note: These figures may differ from those published previously because the Unit is still identifying cases from previous years.

Source: UK CJD Surveillance Unit

epidemiology of CJD in the UK, with particular attention paid to occupation and eating habits; the data for 1995 do not provide conclusive evidence of any change in CJD attributable to bovine spongiform encephalopathy (BSE).

During 1995, there were 43 deaths from CJD and Gerstmann-Straussler-Scheinker syndrome (see Table 9.1). The number of sporadic cases (36) represents a decrease on the 1994 figure of 53 cases, although this finding remains provisional until the 1995 data are finalised. The cases recorded included a fourth case in a farmer, the first in a teenager, and two in individuals aged 29 and 30 years; the latter three cases also have unusual clinicopathological features. The findings in these cases and in a further seven other similar ones (either still alive or who died in early 1996, including a second case in a teenager) will be reported in Spring 1996[1] (see pages 2-3). Surveillance will need to continue for some years in view of the potentially prolonged incubation period of CJD.

Reference

1. Will RG, Ironside JW, Zeider M et al. A new variant of Creutzfeldt-Jakob disease in the UK. *Lancet* (in press).

(k) Bioethics

(i) Research ethics committees

In 1991, each District Health Authority was required to establish a Local Research Ethics Committee (LREC). Subsequent initiatives have addressed training, quality standards and options to streamline the process of ethical approval for health-related multi-centre research. Working closely with a consultative group convened by the Chief Medical Officer, DH developed proposals for wider consultation to establish a Multi-centre Research Ethics Committee (MREC) in each health region. An MREC would advise nationally, not just within its host region, on the science and general ethics of the research protocols it considered. LRECs would continue to advise on local acceptability.

The Department's standards framework for LRECs[1] and further information on standard operating procedures for LRECs[2] were widely used to promote nationally consistent good practice, to clarify LRECs' objectives, and to identify training needs and scope for improvement through managerial action.

(ii) Bioethics in Europe

The Council of Europe's Steering Committee on Bioethics (CDBI) is charged with studying the impact of progress in biomedical sciences on law, ethics and human rights. A draft framework Bioethics Convention was issued for consultation in July 1994 and the CDBI considered comments received in 1995. This work should be completed during 1996.

(iii)   Human genetics

Last year's Report[3] recorded the start of an inquiry into human genetics by the House of Commons Select Committee on Science and Technology. The Select Committee's report[4] was published in July, and examined genetic research, diagnosis and screening, gene therapy, patenting and the social issues raised by developments in genetics. The Government was due to respond to this report early in 1996.

(iv)   Human Fertilisation and Embryology Authority

The Human Fertilisation and Embryology Authority (HFEA), currently chaired by Mrs Ruth Deech, was established by the Human Fertilisation and Embryology Act 1990[5,6]. It is responsible for the regulation of clinical practice that involves the keeping of human embryos outwith the woman's body, the donation and cryopreservation of gametes (eggs and sperm), and research on embryos. Regulation is through licensing and a code of practice[7].

During 1995, after consultation on publishing the success rates for treatment by donor insemination (DI) and in-vitro fertilisation (IVF) for individual licensed centres, the HFEA published *The patients' guide to DI and IVF clinics*[8]. The Authority prepared a report to UK Health Ministers on the statutory storage period for frozen embryos, after taking account of a wide range of views.

(v)   Gene Therapy Advisory Committee

The Gene Therapy Advisory Committee (GTAC) met three times during 1995 and received six protocols for review. The Committee was content, in principle, for three protocols for gene therapy research in human beings to proceed; two protocols were still under consideration at the end of the year. The remaining protocol was withdrawn at the request of the proposers, and is expected to be resubmitted during 1996.

In total, since 1993, GTAC and its predecessor, the Clothier Committee, have completed the review of research protocols for the following diseases: severe combined immunodeficiency (1), cystic fibrosis (4), malignant melanoma (2), lymphoma (2), neuroblastoma (1), breast cancer (1), Hurler's syndrome (1) and cancer of the cervix (1). In addition, protocols have been submitted for studies in neck and head cancer and in acute myeloid leukaemia. A total of 55 patients have been recruited in nine trials that involve gene transfers.

During 1995, GTAC published a booklet[9] which provides detailed advice for principal investigators and clinicians on writing information leaflets to patients who participate in gene therapy research.

(vi)   Protection and use of patient information

The Department prepared the first detailed guidance for the NHS on the protection and use of patient information for publication in Spring 1996[10]. This guidance will emphasise the legal duty of all NHS bodies and staff to protect patient confidentiality while recognising that, for the NHS to function effectively in everyone's interests, some patient information will be needed for a number of purposes other than care or treatment (such as for training, audit and planning purposes). The arrangements will be underpinned by patients being properly informed of how personal information, anonymised wherever possible, may be used. As far as possible the guidance takes account of the EU Directive on Data Protection, adopted during 1995 for implementation by 1998.

References

1. Department of Health. *Standards for Local Research Ethics Committees: a framework for ethical review.* London: Department of Health, 1994.
2. Bendall C. *Standard operating procedures for Local Research Ethics Committees.* London: Department of Health, 1994.
3. Department of Health. *On the State of the Public Health: the annual report of the Chief Medical Officer of the Department of Health for the year 1994.* London: HMSO, 1995; 221.
4. House of Commons Select Committee on Science and Technology. *Human genetics: the science and its consequences.* London: HMSO, 1995.
5. *The Human Fertilisation and Embryology Act 1990.* London: HMSO, 1990.
6. *The Human Fertilisation and Embryology Act 1990 (Commencement no. 2 and Transitional Provision) Order 1991.* London: HMSO, 1991 (Statutory Instrument: SI 1991 no. 480 c.10).
7. Human Fertilisation and Embryology Authority. *Code of practice (second revision, December 1995).* London: Human Fertilisation and Embryology Authority, 1995.
8. Human Fertilisation and Embryology Authority. *The patients' guide to DI and IVF clinics.* London: Human Fertilisation and Embryology Authority, 1995.
9. Gene Therapy Advisory Committee. *Writing information leaflets for patients participating in gene therapy research.* London: Department of Health, 1995.
10. Department of Health. *The protection and use of patient information.* London: Department of Health (in press).

(l) Complaints

March saw the publication of DH's plans for a new simplified NHS complaints procedure, *Acting on complaints*[1]. This followed extensive consultation on recommendations in *Being heard*[2], the report of the independent committee which the then Secretary of State for Health had appointed to review NHS complaints arrangements.

The new complaints arrangements will be brought into use on 1 April 1996. They will focus on local resolution, where the service provider (eg, the hospital or GP) will try to resolve the complaint, in most cases on an informal basis and as quickly as possible, but ensuring a thorough response. If the matter is not resolved at this stage, an independent review will involve further consideration of the complaint by a non-executive director of the NHS Trust or health authority in consultation with an independent lay person. This may result in the establishment of an independent panel with a majority of independent members, or further action by the service provider to resolve the matter.

If they are not satisfied with the response from the NHS, complainants may refer the matter to the Health Service Commissioner. The Government introduced a Bill to Parliament on 29 November to widen the Commissioner's jurisdiction to include complaints about matters arising from the exercise of clinical judgment and about family health services.

References

1. Department of Health. *Acting on complaints: the Government's proposals in response to 'Being heard', the report of a review committee on NHS complaints procedures.* Wetherby (West Yorkshire): Department of Health, 1995 (Executive Letter: EL(95)37).
2. Department of Health. *Being heard: the report of a review committee on NHS complaints procedures.* Leeds: Department of Health, 1994. Chair: Professor Alan Wilson.

(m)   Research and development

The Department's research and development (R&D) strategy promotes strong links with the science base and with other major research funders. A national forum has been established to establish closer working links between research interests in the NHS and elsewhere, including the Research Councils, the Association of Medical Research Charities, industry and universities (see page 130).

Collaboration between UK Health Departments and the Medical Research Council (MRC) is formalised in a Concordat which is currently being reviewed. Concordats have also been established with the Engineering and Physical Sciences Research Council and with the Biotechnology and Biological Sciences Research Council. An Agreement is in place with the Economic and Social Research Council.

DH, with the MRC, has helped to shape the EU's Biomedicine and Health Research Programme (BIOMED) within the Fourth Framework Programme for Research and Technological Development (FP4). The Department also has an interest in other related FP4 components, including the telematics programme and the radiation protection programme in EURATOM. The Department is involved in consultation to establish UK views on priorities for the Fifth Framework Programme (FP5), which will start in 1999.

(n)   Use of information technology in clinical care

The NHS information management and technology (IM&T) strategy is directed towards the use of information technology as an aid to delivery of effective and efficient health care. It has a number of key programmes - such as NHS-wide networking and administrative registers - on which work continued during the year; taken together, these programmes will provide the necessary infrastructure to support health care in the future. During 1995, a number of important developments were seen.

Ways to support clinical effectiveness with IM&T have been examined. Plans were made to make national and international research on clinical effectiveness and other areas available via the NHS-wide network during 1996-97.

There are real benefits to clinicians if appropriate information can be made available at the point of care. During the year, the PRODIGY project has developed computer-aided decision support for general practitioner (GP) prescribing. Prescribing benefits have also been seen during work on the electronic patient record project at the Wirral and Burton NHS Trusts.

Practical experience of integrating information by use of clinical workstations has been gained during a project run at the Horizon, Bethlem and Maudsley, and Winchester NHS Trusts. This integrated clinical workstation project, with the electronic patient record project, addressed many of the complex cultural and technical issues that underlie the use of information technology to support clinical care.

The IM&T training programme for clinicians has made good progress in the development of links with clinical training facilities, and a database of up-to-date information on sources of relevant IM&T training has been produced. A joint working group was established with the council of medical school deans, and a workshop for all UK medical schools was held in December. Initiatives to support good quality clinical coding of information have been promoted by the National Centre for Coding and Classification (see page 135).

The 'Patients not paper' efficiency scrutiny[1] highlighted the need to reduce paperwork flowing into and out of general practices and stressed that best use of IM&T was needed to achieve this. Work continued to ensure that all GPs will be linked via the NHS-wide network to health authorities and providers of health care. This linkage will support the development of a primary care-led NHS.

GP records have potentially the richest source of morbidity and health data in the NHS. Work continued to address the necessary recording standards and confidentiality policies that are needed before such data can be shared and used to support achievement of Health of the Nation targets[2] and locality purchasing.

Security and confidentiality is a major ethical concern which also has an important technical dimension. Guidance on NHS-wide networking security has been issued[3], and discussions continued with professional bodies to agree ways to achieve the secure sharing of clinical information between appropriate professionals (see page 215).

Work progressed on health care resource groupings for use in costing, contracting and internal resource management. The use of health benefit groupings for analysis of epidemiological data to assist purchasers of health care to define their needs continued.

The Read Code project (see page 135) has created an agreed computerised health care thesaurus of clinical terms after work which involved over 55 specialty working groups and over 2,000 clinicians; version 3 of the Code was released in April. Transition to the International Classification of Diseases version 10 (ICD-10) for the coding of hospital diagnoses was made successfully in April. Introduction of the new NHS number (starting with newborn babies) began in December. The transmission of electronic messages that use nationally agreed standards began in a number of key areas - such as referral and discharge summaries, and radiology and pathology test requests and results.

As the national IM&T infrastructure develops, so the potential benefits from the use of information technology to support the provision of health care to individual patients can be more fully realised.

References

1. NHS Executive. *Patients not paper: report of the efficiency scrutiny into bureaucracy in general practice.* Wetherby (West Yorkshire): Department of Health, 1995.
2. Department of Health. *The Health of the Nation: a strategy for health in England.* London: HMSO, 1992 (Cm. 1986).
3. Information Management Group, NHS Executive. *NHS-wide networking programme: NHS-wide networking security project: security guide for IM&T specialists.* Wetherby (West Yorkshire): Department of Health, 1995 (IMG E5216).

(o)   Dental health

(i)   *Dental health of the nation*

The National Diet and Nutrition Survey of children aged $1^1/_2$ to $4^1/_2$ years was published in March (see also page 70)[1]. Among the findings of the dental survey were:

—   83% of children in this age-group were caries-free;

—   most of the dental decay present in the other 17% was untreated;

—   children who started having their teeth brushed or who were brushing their own teeth before the age of one year were significantly less likely to have experience of dental decay than those who started toothbrushing later;

—   87% of children had been fed from bottles at some time, and a higher proportion of those aged $1^1/_2$-$2^1/_2$ and $2^1/_2$-$3^1/_2$ years, who had a drink in bed every night, had decay experience than of those who only occasionally or never had a drink in bed; *and*

—   among those children who consumed sugar confectionery on most days of the week or more often, the proportion with tooth decay was almost double that among those who consumed sugar confectionery less frequently. Frequent consumption of carbonated drinks was also related to experience of dental decay.

The results of this survey also confirm the importance of water fluoridation, effective health education and continued emphasis on achieving and maintaining oral health in childhood if the trend of improved oral health is to be maintained.

Surveys conducted by health authorities in 1994-95 show a continued improvement in the dental health of 14-year-olds, with an overall reduction in decay experience of 20% compared with four years ago. However, wide regional variations remain and there is an apparent increase in the amount of unrestored decay (where it has occurred) in this age-group.

In November, building on the recommendations in its oral health strategy, DH convened a National Advisory Group for the Screening of Oral Cancer (NAGSOC). Chaired by the Chief Dental Officer, the Group will evaluate the methods presently used by general dental practitioners when they screen for oral cancer. The NAGSOC will also consider what information practitioners need to screen effectively in the future.

(ii)   General dental services

The period of formal consultation on the Government's Green Paper *Improving NHS dentistry*[2] ended on 1 November 1994. The Government listened carefully to the views of the profession. Proposals to improve NHS dentistry were announced by Mr Gerald Malone, the Minister for Health, in a Parliamentary answer on 5 April. Mr Malone said that the statement underpinned the Government's commitment to NHS dentistry. The reforms aimed to provide a framework for continuing improvement in oral health, and reinforced the priority of the oral health of children. They would ensure the continued availability of NHS dentistry in all parts of the UK, and end uncertainty in the dental profession.

The reforms will be introduced in two phases: there will be immediate action to deliver improvements to the current system and continued work on the long-term reform of the structure of NHS dentistry.

Reform of the current system will include improvements to child capitation by relating payments to dentists to disease levels in children most at need. The continuing care relationship between dentists and patients will remain, but changes to the current flat-rate system of continuing care payments will provide better value for taxpayers' money. In adult care, more rigorous prior approval procedures for monitoring treatment will be introduced to ensure that the general dental service (GDS) provides only those treatments which are clinically essential and for which there is no clinically acceptable, less costly alternative.

In the longer term, the Government aims to introduce a system of local contracts between health authorities and dental practices similar to that which operates in other parts of the health service. This system will be carefully piloted and thoroughly evaluated before a decision would be taken on nationwide introduction. Primary legislation will be sought to set up pilot schemes.

Some dentists are still limiting their commitment to NHS dentistry, as they have always been able to do. Monitoring indicates that although general dental services are maintained in most areas, there are local pockets where there are shortages of NHS dentists which, in some instances, can lead to patients travelling further for treatment than they might wish.

(iii)	*Community dental services*

The community dental service (CDS) retains responsibility for monitoring the dental health of the population (for example, by undertaking surveys to investigate the disease trends of oral disease and to establish attitudes to and use of dental services), and for dental health education and preventive programmes. Additionally, the service is responsible for the provision of facilities for a full range of treatment to patients who have experienced difficulty in obtaining treatment in the GDS, or for whom there is evidence that they would not otherwise seek treatment from the GDS.

One component of the Government's package to improve NHS dentistry, announced on 5 April, was to develop the role of the CDS to meet the needs of patients in areas of the country where there is difficulty in obtaining NHS treatment under the GDS.

A comparative evaluation of the work of senior dental officers and associate specialists (dental) found similar levels of responsibility held by holders of the two posts. The UK Health Departments and the British Dental Association, in joint evidence presented to the Review Body on Doctors' and Dentists' Remuneration, agreed that this should be recognised by a closer alignment of the salary scales for these two groups.

It had been a concern to the profession that no non-academic consultants in dental public health were receiving distinction awards; agreement was reached to include consultants in dental public health in an NHS-wide scheme to replace the 'C' award system with a scheme of up to five discretionary points.

(iv)	*Hospital dental services*

The number of hospital dentists in England rose by 1.5% from 1,270 to 1,289 between September 1993 and September 1994. In September 1994, there were 435 consultants in post, an increase of 3.1% over the previous year. The number of senior registrars fell from 112 to 101 and the number of senior house officers rose from 294 to 324. (Figures given refer to whole-time equivalent posts.)

In 1994/95, there was a fall in new outpatient referrals to consultant clinics of 1.5% compared with 1993/94. In oral surgery, referrals rose by 0.4% from 400,123 to 401,552. Referrals in orthodontics fell by 0.2% from 105,709 to 105,513. In restorative dentistry, referrals fell by 4.9% from 48,126 to 45,762, and referrals in paediatric dentistry fell by 30.7% from 24,193 to 16,754. Over the same period, repeat attendances at outpatient clinics fell by 6.1%. Repeat attendances in oral surgery fell by 5.3% from 721,494 to 683,230, and in orthodontics repeat attendances fell by 4.1% from 667,859 to 640,534. Repeat attendances in restorative dentistry fell by 10.4% from 352,003 to 315,234, and in paediatric dentistry they fell by 12.2% from 74,237 to 65,201.

(v)   Continuing education and training for dentists

There were 517 trainees in 48 regionally based vocational training schemes on 1 October. The Committee for Continuing Education and Training identified the following priority areas for the training of general dental practitioners in 1994/95: supporting the oral health strategy; 'hands-on' courses; sedation techniques; pain control and the management of anxious patients; the management of elderly or disabled patients and those with special needs; the Nutrition Task Force's curriculum for health care professionals; courses to reinforce distance learning programmes; the training of trainers, advisers and examiners; research techniques relevant to general dental practice; training practice staff; and courses to promote peer review and clinical audit in general dental practice. These courses are arranged by postgraduate dental deans or directors of dental education and funded by DH under the provisions of Section 63 of the Health Services and Public Health Act 1968[3].

During 1995, DH continued to fund the production and distribution of distance learning material for general dental practitioners, including a teaching video on oral radiography and a range of computer-assisted learning programmes.

(vi)   Dental research

Diet and oral health

As part of the National Diet and Nutrition Survey programme, a team from the Universities of Birmingham and Newcastle-upon-Tyne and the Office of Population Censuses and Surveys (OPCS, to become part of the Office for National Statistics in 1996) was commissioned to conduct a survey on the condition and function of oral tissues of a sample of about 2,000 subjects aged 4 to 18 years, and to relate their findings to the diet and nutritional status of these subjects.

Also as part of this programme, the field work for a similar survey of subjects aged 65 years and over was completed in 1995; a report is expected in 1997. A report of findings in children aged $1^1/_2$-$4^1/_2$years was published in March (see page 219).

NHS research and development programme

A co-ordinated NHS Research and Development programme for primary dental care was announced in June[4]. The programme resulted from a review conducted on behalf of the Department by the former Mersey Regional Health Authority (RHA), in which priority areas were identified and ranked. These ranged from the accessibility and availability of services to the occupational health of dental personnel. The North West RHA R&D Directorate are managing the programme.

Children's dental health under the GDS capitation scheme

Commissioned reports from the Universities of Birmingham and Manchester were received by the Department. These studies indicate that regional and ethnic differences in dental caries experience persist; that the provision of intervention treatments has reduced; and that oral hygiene and dietary advice has increased since the capitation scheme was introduced. Caries experience, particularly in deciduous teeth, was still too high.

References

1. Gregory JR, Collins DL, Davies PSW, Hughes JM, Clarke PC, Hinds K. *National Diet and Nutrition Survey: children aged $1^1/2$ to $4^1/2$ years: vol. 2: report of the dental survey.* London: HMSO, 1995.
2. Department of Health. *Improving NHS dentistry.* London: HMSO, 1994 (Cm. 2625).
3. *The Health Services and Public Health Act 1968.* London: HMSO, 1968.
4. Department of Health. *Dental specialisation will develop dentists' skills, says Gerald Malone.* London: Department of Health, 1995 (Press Release: H95/272).

CHAPTER 10

INTERNATIONAL HEALTH

(a)   England, Europe and health

Many of the health challenges encountered in England and the United Kingdom (UK) as a whole are also found in the rest of Europe; diseases have little respect for national boundaries. The pace of technological advance, ageing populations and rising expectations are leading to growing demands on health care services throughout Europe and beyond. The challenges of drug dependence and other lifestyle-related health problems are common to many countries.

The opportunity to work together on common problems within the European Community (EC), and in international bodies such as the World Health Organization (WHO) and the Council of Europe, brings great benefits. The UK has much expertise to offer, but can also benefit greatly from the knowledge of others, the insight provided by international comparisons, and the greater resources that international co-operation can bring into play.

Nowhere can be insulated from the changes taking place. Political change in Central and Eastern Europe has opened up the prospect of much greater freedom of movement, but has also produced dislocation in which old diseases have re-emerged and health care has deteriorated. Migration to the EC has increased rapidly, bringing groups who have distinct health needs and present new challenges to the public health systems of host countries.

(i)   The European Union

The Council of Health Ministers

The Council of Ministers is a key decision-making body of the EC, in which all Member States are represented. Councils of Ministers with particular responsibilities, such as health, meet regularly to deal with relevant EC business.

In 1995, the Health Council held general meetings on 2 June and 30 November. These took forward proposals for EC action in line with the Framework for Action in the Field of Public Health published in November 1993[1]. The November Health Council agreed final decisions on proposed programmes on AIDS and certain other communicable diseases, cancer, and health promotion. Formal adoption of these programmes, and one on drug dependence, by the Health Council and the European Parliament are expected in 1996.

High Level Committee on Health

The High Level Committee on Health, which generally meets twice a year, is composed of representatives of each Member State. Its role is to provide advice to the European Commission and the Health Council on the appropriateness of, and need for, proposals for Community action; it has no executive powers. In 1995, the Commission proposed that the Committee, which had been operating informally since 1991, should be given formal status. Work to develop its new status is still in progress. During 1995, the Committee considered a number of important and topical issues, including future work in the field of public health research and the integration of public health requirements across the policies of the EC.

Meetings of European Chief Medical Officers

The Chief Medical Officers of the Member States meet informally twice a year to exchange professional views on Community health policy, and on relevant WHO and Council of Europe programmes. Their meetings, which are attended by representatives of the WHO and the Council of Europe, provide an ideal opportunity to promote closer collaboration between the EC, the WHO and the Council of Europe.

Other European Community programmes

In October 1995, the European Commission published its proposal on health monitoring, and agreement on a common position is expected at the Health Council meeting in May 1996. Further proposals on pollution-related illnesses, accidents and injuries, and rare diseases are also expected during 1996.

The Council of Ministers and the European Parliament formally adopted the Data Protection Directive on 24 October 1995. The latest date for introduction of provisions to give effect to the Directive in the UK is 24 October 1998. The Department of Health (DH) will begin work on an implementation strategy in 1996.

During 1995, there was continued EC activity related to: health of adolescents (see page 72); health of women (see page 73); health of men (see page 73); food safety and surveillance (see page 180); emerging infectious diseases (see page 181); environment and health (see page 186); postgraduate and specialist medical education (see page 195); pharmaceutical marketing authorisation (see page 204); medical devices (see page 205); bioethics (see page 214); and research and technological development (see page 217).

Free movement of people

Health professionals

The number of health professionals from other Member States of the European Economic Area (EEA) working in the UK is small and most come for short periods to gain experience. In 1995, 1,803 doctors with qualifications from other Member States obtained full registration with the General Medical Council, 332 dentists with the General Dental Council, 28 pharmacists with the Royal

Pharmaceutical Society of Great Britain, 759 nurses and 33 midwives with the UK Central Council of Nursing, Midwifery and Health Visiting, and 411 persons with the Council for the Professions Supplementary to Medicine (comprising 10 chiropodists, 81 occupational therapists, 37 dietitians, 197 physiotherapists, 73 radiographers, 2 orthoptists and 11 medical laboratory scientific officers).

Patients

EC Social Security Regulation 1408/71 continued to operate satisfactorily, co-ordinating health care cover for people moving between EEA Member States. The main categories covered were temporary visitors, detached workers and pensioners transferring their residence to another Member State. In 1995, 644 applications by UK patients for referral to other Member States specifically for treatment of pre-existing conditions were approved by DH. About 318 citizens of other Member States were treated in the UK on the same basis.

EC/WHO/Council of Europe

Close co-operation between the EC, the WHO and the Council of Europe continued during 1995. Examples of collaboration include support for the establishment of the joint and co-sponsored United Nations (UN) programme on HIV/AIDS (UNAIDS); continued co-operation on the safety of blood and blood products; and the joint WHO/EC/Council of Europe European Network of Health Promoting Schools project. Thirty countries have now joined this Network and some 300,000 pupils from more than 400 schools are already participating in exciting new health promotion pilot schemes. A further 1,600 schools are linked to the Network, exchanging views and ideas to assist the development of health promotion for young people.

(ii)   Council of Europe

During 1995, the Council's European Health Committee took forward work on organ transplantation, blood, patients' rights, access to treatment, systems for assessing quality of service, and a co-ordinated research study on the organisation of health services for elderly people in institutional care.

The Council adopted recommendations on the protection of the health of donors and recipients of blood and blood products (reaffirming the principle of voluntary and non-remunerated blood, plasma and cell donation); on the preparation, use and quality assurance of blood components; and on nursing research (recommending that Governments should implement measures to identify needs, strategies and priorities in nursing research).

A super-urgent liver exchange network was established on an experimental basis between France, Italy and Switzerland. Information is being gathered on transplant criteria in Member States and on the legal and bioethical aspects of xenotransplantation.

(iii)   Relations with Central and Eastern Europe

By the end of 1995, the European Union (EU) had concluded 'Europe Agreements' with nine Central and Eastern European Countries - Bulgaria, the Czech Republic, Estonia, Hungary, Latvia, Lithuania, Poland, Romania and Slovakia - and six of these (with Bulgaria, the Czech Republic, Hungary, Poland, Romania and Slovakia) were in force.   The agreements are intended to strengthen economic links by enabling free trade for industrial products and are designed to lead towards EU membership.   Poland and Hungary had already applied for full membership of the EU in 1994, and a further six countries did so during 1995; the Czech Republic is expected to follow suit early in 1996.

To assist Central and Eastern European countries in their preparation for future accession, the European Commission published a White Paper[2] in May 1995, setting out its view of the legislation which they should adopt to prepare themselves for participation in the Single European Market.   The White Paper emphasised the role of the EC's PHARE programme (Poland and Hungary Assistance for Economic Restructuring) in providing funds to countries hoping for EU membership.   This funding will in the future concentrate on assistance in preparing for participation in the single market.

Partnership and co-operation agreements were also concluded in 1995 with several countries of the former Soviet Union - Belarus, Kazakhstan, Kyrgyzstan, Russia, and the Ukraine.   Similar agreements with Armenia, Azerbaijan and Georgia are expected to be signed during 1996.   Financial support for restructuring in these countries continued to be provided by the TACIS programme (Technical Assistance to the Commonwealth of Independent States).

DH continued to support exchange visits by specialists under the UK's Health Co-operation Agreements with Bulgaria, Hungary, Poland, Romania, Russia and the Czech and Slovak Republics.

References

1.   Commission of the European Communities. *Commission communication on the framework for action in the field of public health.* Luxembourg: Office for Official Publications of the European Communities, 1993 (COM(93); 559 final).
2.   Commission of the European Communities. *White Paper: preparation of the associated countries of Central and Eastern Europe for integration into the internal market of the Union.* Luxembourg: Office for Official Publications of the European Communities, 1995 (COM(95); 163 final).

(b)   The Commonwealth

The 11th triennial Commonwealth Health Ministers' Meeting was held in Cape Town in December.   This was the first ministerial meeting to be held in South Africa since its readmission to the Commonwealth; 32 countries were represented, together with the WHO, the UN Children's Fund and seven Non-Governmental Organisations.   The British delegation was led by Baroness Cumberlege, Parliamentary Under Secretary of State for Health in the House of Lords, supported by the Chief Medical and Nursing Officers.

The theme for the meeting, 'Women and Health', was timely as it followed a number of international conferences on women's health, including the Fourth World Conference on Women in Beijing in September. At the opening ceremony, Dr Nkosazana Zuma, the South African Health Minister, challenged her colleagues to co-operate to transform gender discrimination in the same way that South Africa had transformed itself following the abolition of apartheid.

The agenda was considered in two parts. One committee, chaired by Baroness Cumberlege, addressed issues under the broad heading of 'Women for health', including the major role of women in the provision of informal care and their limited contribution to national policy formation. Of particular interest was the report on the Commonwealth Action Plan for Nursing and Midwifery, prepared by a Steering Group chaired by the Chief Nursing Officer. Health Ministers made a number of recommendations to Governments designed to enhance the role of women in policy formulation and decision-making, and to strengthen the role of nurses and midwives. The other committee addressed issues under the broad heading of 'Health for women', including violence against women, reproductive and sexual health, HIV/AIDS, non-communicable diseases, and researching, promoting and teaching women's health; it also agreed recommendations for further action.

Health Ministers recommended that a Technical Support Group should be established to help the Commonwealth Secretariat, in its advocacy, brokerage and catalytic role, to take forward these recommendations for action. Ministers agreed to monitor progress closely at their annual meetings immediately before the World Health Assembly, and at the 12th Commonwealth Health Ministers' Meeting in 1998.

(c)   World Health Organization

(i)   *European Regional Committee*

The 45th session of the European Regional Committee was held in Jerusalem in September; the Chief Medical Officer led the UK delegation. With a budget allocation some £6.5 million less than expected and planned for, the Region faced difficult decisions at a time when there was clear evidence of an increasing incidence of communicable diseases - particularly cholera, diphtheria, polio and tuberculosis. The countries mainly affected are those in Central and Eastern Europe, especially some of the Newly Independent States of the former Soviet Union. EUROHEALTH, the Region's top priority programme, is directed at these countries and the UK played a major role in building support for a re-ordering of priorities within the programme to address the growing problem of communicable diseases. The UK was elected as one of the Region's nominees to the Executive Board of WHO and, subject to ratification by the World Health Assembly, the Chief Medical Officer will be a member of that Board from May 1996.

Separately from the formal business of the meeting, the Chief Medical Officer renewed the plan of co-operation under the Health Co-operation Agreement with Romania.

(ii)   Executive Board

In January, the Chief Medical Officer attended the 95th session of the WHO Executive Board in Geneva. The main item considered was the draft programme budget for the 1996-97 biennium. The Board adopted a resolution urging the Director General to reallocate at least 5% of the budget to priority areas such as the prevention, control and eradication of specific communicable diseases; reproductive health, women's health and family health; promotion of primary care including essential drugs, vaccines and nutrition; and promotion of environmental health. Governing bodies, procurement, staff costs and administrative services were identified as areas from which resources might be diverted. The Board was satisfied with progress towards the implementation of recommendations for reform of the organisation in response to global change, but identified areas on which further work was required.

Immediately before the Board meeting, the Chief Medical Officer attended the first meeting of the Administration, Budget and Finance Committee - one of two sub-committees set up following acceptance of recommendations on reforming the WHO in response to global change.

The Executive Board held its 96th session immediately after the World Health Assembly in May. The main item considered was the implementation of the Assembly's resolutions on the WHO budget. It was agreed to consider changes to the constitution at the next Executive Board meeting in January 1996.

(iii)   World Health Assembly

The 48th World Health Assembly, the annual meeting of the Member States of the WHO, took place in Geneva in May. The UK delegation was led by Mrs Virginia Bottomley, the then Secretary of State for Health, and included the Chief Medical Officer, the Chief Nursing Officer, and officials from DH, the Overseas Development Administration and the UK Mission in Geneva.

In her address to the plenary session, Mrs Bottomley spoke of progress on the Health of the Nation initiative. She stressed the need for health care resources to be allocated according to priorities that took careful account of an assessment of health needs, and for Governments to assess the health impact of all their policies.

The main decision taken at the Assembly was the setting of the WHO budget for the 1996-97 biennium. Member States agreed a zero-rate-of-growth budget, with a 2.5% increase to take account of global inflation and international currency fluctuations.

Other resolutions covered a wide range of issues including a global strategy on reproductive health, the control of new and emerging communicable diseases, and a request to the Executive Board to consider an international strategy for tobacco control. Member States were satisfied with progress on the reform of the WHO but noted areas where further work was required.

During the Assembly the first World Health Report was published in response to a recommendation of the Working Group on WHO's response to change, chaired by the Chief Medical Officer. Based on the theme 'Bridging the gaps', it combined an assessment of world health status with a report on WHO activities, highlighting global inequalities in health and the major impact of poverty on morbidity and mortality.

APPENDIX

Appendix Tables and their content

Appendix Table 1: *Population age and sex structure, England, mid-1995, and changes by age, 1981-91, 1991-92, 1992-93, 1993-94 and 1994-95.*

This Table is described in Chapter 1 (see page 47).

Appendix Tables 2A and 2B: *Five main causes of death for males and females at different ages, England, 1994 (A) and 1995 (B).*

This Table is presented for both 1994 and 1995. It contrasts the main causes of death in different age-groups for males and females alike. The results for 1994 and 1995 are very similar.

It should be noted that the rankings are dependent upon how diseases are grouped. The International Classification of Diseases (ICD) is divided into 17 broad chapters, covering different types of diseases - for example respiratory diseases. Within these chapters, individual diseases or groups of diseases are given a 3-digit code, which in most cases can be further broken down into 4-digit codes. For the purposes of producing these Tables, distinct diseases have been used in most cases - vague remainder categories have been avoided, even if there were a higher number of deaths, in order to make the data more meaningful and useful. However, for the 1-14 years age-group, where the numbers of deaths are very small, the rankings are based on whole chapters of the ICD.

At the age of 35 years and over, the major burden of mortality derives from circulatory disease and malignant neoplasms. At ages over 74 years, respiratory diseases also contribute strongly. At ages 15-34 years, suicide and undetermined injury and motor vehicle traffic accidents are the leading causes of death for males and females alike. The leading cause of death among children is external causes of injury and poisoning (mostly accidents).

The 1993 data presented in last year's Report[1] were recalculated using the above method. The patterns were the same as for 1994 and 1995.

Appendix Tables 3A and 3B: *Relative mortality from various conditions when presented as numbers of deaths and future years of 'working life' lost, England and Wales, 1994 (A) and 1995 (B).*

This Table is presented for both 1994 and 1995. The total number of deaths at all ages attributed to selected causes are given. The percentage distribution of deaths demonstrates the major impact of circulatory disease and cancer in both sexes. The figures for 1994 and 1995 are very similar. In 1995, over 80% of deaths occurred at the age of 65 years and over.

Years of 'working life' lost between the ages of 15 and 64 years indicate the impact of various causes of death occurring at younger ages. For this table, a death occurring under the age of 15 years accounts for the loss of the full 50-year period between the ages of 15 and 64 years, whereas a death at age 60 years contributes a loss of only 5 years of 'working life'. Thus weight is given to the age at death as well as the number of deaths, and emphasis is given to the burden of deaths occurring at younger ages.

For males, although circulatory disease and cancer still contribute substantially to loss of 'working life', other causes become more prominent. These include accidents and suicide and undetermined injury, and also those deaths occurring early in life - particularly infant deaths, which account for about 15% of years of 'working life' lost.

For females, the total years of future 'working life' lost from all causes combined is much less than for males, reflecting considerably lower death rates in females. Cancer - particularly of the breast, cervix, uterus and ovary - is a major contributor to loss of life in females aged under 65 years. In 1995, cancer accounted for 23% of all female deaths, but 40% of years of 'working life' lost. By contrast, although causing 43% of the total number of deaths, circulatory disease accounted for only 16% of the years of 'working life' lost. In other respects, the pattern is broadly similar to that for males, although accidents and suicide account for a smaller proportion of deaths among females.

The 1993 data presented in last year's Report were recalculated. The results were very similar except for a reduction in the years of 'working life' lost from respiratory diseases and sudden infant death syndrome. However, the revised results obtained for 1993 were very similar to those presented here for 1994 and 1995.

Appendix Table 4: *Trends in 'avoidable' deaths, England, 1979-95.*

The concept of 'avoidable' deaths was discussed in detail in the Report of 1987[2]. These indicators - developed in this country by Professor Walter Holland and his colleagues[3] - have been chosen to identify selected causes of mortality amenable to health service intervention, either preventive or curative. They might best be called 'potentially avoidable' deaths as, while it might not be possible to prevent every death deemed avoidable, it is expected that a substantial proportion could be prevented. The indicators are now published as part of the Public Health Common Data Set.

The Table presents recent secular trends of nine categories of 'avoidable' deaths. The data are presented as age-standardised mortality ratios, which adjust for differences in the age structure in the years compared. During the period 1979-95, substantial declines are evident in all of the categories presented. The age-standardised mortality ratio for all 'avoidable' deaths combined has fallen by 50% since 1979.

Appendix Table 5: *Live births, stillbirths, infant mortality and abortions, England, 1960, 1970, 1975-95.*

Trends are discussed in Chapter 1 (see page 58).

Appendix Table 6: *Congenital anomalies, England, 1985, 1990, 1994 and 1995.*

This Table shows the numbers of babies notified with selected congenital anomalies. In the past, the Table referred to the number of mentions of selected anomalies, but this was difficult to interpret as a baby can have more than one congenital anomaly. The data for 1985, 1990 and 1994 have been re-calculated to enable comparisons over time, but it should be noted (see Chapter 1, page 60) that changes to the notification list in January 1990 affected the following groups: ear and eye malformations, cardiovascular malformations and talipes.

Appendix Table 7: *Cancer registrations by age and site, males, England and Wales, 1991.*

The Table indicates the distribution of cancer registrations in men at different ages. At all ages combined, cancers of the lung, large intestine (including rectum) and prostate account for half of the registrations. In childhood, a high proportion of cancers are attributable to leukaemias, lymphomas, tumours of the central nervous system, and embryonic tumours such as neuroblastomas and retinoblastomas. At older ages, cancer of the lung is the major cause registered. In the oldest age-group presented (85 years and over), prostate cancer accounts for slightly more registrations than lung cancer.

Appendix Table 8: *Cancer registrations by age and site, females, England and Wales, 1991.*

In childhood, the pattern of female cancers is broadly similar to that in males. However, in the 25-44 years age-group cancers of the breast (41%) and cervix (17%) predominate. At older ages, breast cancer continues to account for many registrations, although cancers of the lung, large intestine and skin (non-melanoma skin cancers are not included in the Table) also occur in substantial numbers.

Appendix Table 9: *Immunisation uptake, England, 1980-1994/95.*

The information presented in this Table is discussed in Chapter 6 (see page 168).

Appendix Table 10: *Cumulative total of AIDS cases by exposure category, England, to 31 December 1995.*

Recent trends in AIDS cases are discussed in Chapter 6 (see page 156).

Appendix Table 11: *Expectation of life at birth, all-cause death rates and infant mortality, England and European Union countries, circa 1993.*

This Table includes two key overall measures of general health: expectation of life and infant mortality. Recent data are presented for various European countries. Although problems often exist with regard to comparability of data, international comparisons provide an important perspective to the assessment of overall progress. In particular, such comparisons can highlight the scope for improvement and help to stimulate action to achieve progress.

In 1994, average life expectancy at birth in England was 74.5 years in males. Recent figures from our European neighbours ranged from 70.6 years in Portugal to 75.5 years in Sweden. The equivalent figure for females in England was 79.7 years, which compares with a European Union (EU) range from 77.9 years in Denmark and Portugal to 82.3 years in France.

The infant mortality rate is also often used as a key descriptor of the overall health of a country. In 1994, the rate in England was 6.1 per 1,000 live births. This figure was one of the lowest in Europe at that time, contrasting with a rate in Portugal in 1993 of 8.7. Nevertheless, there is no scope for complacency, with lower rates achieved in some other European countries (eg, 5.1 per 1,000 live births in Germany and 4.4 in Finland).

Additional information is presented on the age-standardised all-cause mortality rates for EC countries, with particular reference to deaths occurring under the age of 65 years. For males, the English death rate is well below the EU average and is only bettered by Sweden. However, for women the mortality rate is above the EU average.

All international comparisons need to be made with some caution given possible differences in data collection and recording procedures. However, the indicators presented here are among the most robust for the purpose of comparison.

Appendix Figure 1: *Weekly deaths, England and Wales, 1994 and 1995, and expected deaths, 1995.*

This Figure illustrates the week-by-week registrations of deaths from all causes at ages one year and over for 1995. These are compared with the observed values in 1994 and expected values in 1995. The expected numbers of deaths for 1995 are calculated as an average of the deaths registered in the same week over the previous five-year period, 1990-94.

References

1. Department of Health. *On the State of the Public Health: the annual report of the Chief Medical Officer of the Department of Health for the year 1994.* London: HMSO, 1995; 55, 240.
2. Department of Health and Social Security. *On the State of the Public Health: the annual report of the Chief Medical Officer of the Department of Health and Social Security for the year 1987.* London: HMSO, 1988; 4, 72-82.
3. Charlton JR, Hartley RM, Silver R, Holland WW. Geographical variation in mortality from conditions amenable to medical intervention in England and Wales. *Lancet* 1983; **i:** 691-6.

Table A.1: *Population age and sex structure, England, mid-1995, and changes by age, 1981-91, 1991-92, 1992-93, 1993-94 and 1994-95*

Age (in years)	Resident population at mid-1995 (thousands)			Percentage changes (persons)				
	Persons	Males	Females	1981-91	1991-92	1992-93	1993-94	1994-95
Under 1	615	315	300	10.9	-1.0	-3.6	0.2	-3.1
1-4	2589	1327	1262	15.2	1.2	0.2	-0.4	-0.4
5-15	6844	3513	3331	-13.1	1.2	1.8	1.6	1.0
16-29	9434	4833	4601	4.7	-2.0	-2.5	-2.5	-1.9
30-44	10642	5384	5258	11.5	-0.1	0.8	1.5	1.7
45-64/59*	9870	5492	4378	-0.2	3.0	2.3	1.8	1.4
65/60-74**	5448	1948	3500	-3.2	0.3	0.7	0.5	-1.8
75-84	2568	969	1598	17.6	-1.3	-2.7	-2.4	3.5
85+	893	227	667	49.2	4.7	5.1	3.0	3.4
All ages	48903	24008	24896	3.0	0.4	0.3	0.4	0.4

* 45-64 years for males and 45-59 years for females.
** 65-74 years for males and 60-74 years for females.

Note: Figures may not add precisely to totals due to rounding.

Source: OPCS/ONS

Table A.2A: *Five main causes of death for males and females at different ages (and percentages¹ of all causes of deaths), England, 1994*

Rank	All ages - 1 and over		1-14 years		15-34 years		35-54 years		55-74 years		75 years and over	
	Males	Females	Males	Females	Males	Females	Males	Females	Males	Females	Males	Females
1	410-414 Ischaemic heart disease 28%	410-414 Ischaemic heart disease 22%	E800-E999 External causes of injury and poisoning 30%	E800-999 External causes of injury and poisoning 25%	E950-E959 Suicide and undetermined injury† 24%	E950-959 Suicide and undetermined injury† 12%	410-414 Ischaemic heart disease 24%	174 MN* of female breast 19%	410-414 Ischaemic heart disease 32%	410-414 Ischaemic heart disease 22%	410-414 Ischaemic heart disease 26%	410-414 Ischaemic heart disease 23%
2	430-438 Cerebro-vascular disease 8%	430-438 Cerebro-vascular disease 13%	140-239 Neoplasms 19%	140-239 Neoplasms 17%	E810-E819 Motor vehicle traffic accidents 17%	E810-E819 Motor vehicle traffic accidents 11%	150-159 MN* of digestive organs and peritoneum 9%	179-189 MN* of genito-urinary organs 9%	162 MN* of trachea, bronchus and lung 11%	150-159 MN* of digestive organs and peritoneum 9%	480-486 Pneumonia 11%	430-438 Cerebro-vascular disease 15%
3	162 MN* of trachea, bronchus and lung 8%	480-486 Pneumonia 11%	320-389 Diseases of the nervous system and sense organs 11%	740-759 Congenital anomalies 14%	E850-E869 Accidental poisoning by drugs, medicaments and biologicals 6%	174 MN* of female breast 6%	E950-E959 Suicide and undetermined injury† 7%	150-159 MN* of digestive organs and peritoneum 8%	150-159 MN* of digestive organs and peritoneum 10%	430-438 Cerebro-vascular disease 8%	430-438 Cerebro-vascular disease 11%	480-486 Pneumonia 14%
4	150-159 MN* of digestive organs and peritoneum 8%	150-159 MN* of digestive organs and peritoneum 6%	460-519 Diseases of the respiratory system 10%	320-389 Diseases of the nervous system and sense organs 10%	001-139 Infectious and parasitic diseases 5%	200-208 MN* of lymphatic and haematopoietic tissue 5%	162 MN* of trachea, bronchus and lung 7%	410-414 Ischaemic heart disease 7%	430-438 Cerebro-vascular disease 6%	162 MN* of trachea, bronchus and lung 8%	490-496 Chronic obstructive pulmonary disease and allied conditions 7%	415-429 Diseases of pulmonary circulation and other forms of heart disease 6%
5	480-486 Pneumonia 7%	415-429 Diseases of pulmonary circulation and other forms of heart disease 5%	740-759 Congenital anomalies 9%	460-519 Diseases of the respiratory system 9%	200-208 MN* of lymphatic and haematopoietic tissue 4%	179-189 MN* of genito-urinary organs 5%	430-438 Cerebro-vascular disease 4%	162 MN* of trachea, bronchus and lung 6%	490-496 Chronic obstructive pulmonary disease and allied conditions 6%	174 MN* of female breast 7%	150-159 MN* of digestive organs and peritoneum 6%	150-159 MN* of digestive organs and peritoneum 5%
Remainder	41%	43%	22%	25%	46%	62%	48%	50%	35%	45%	39%	36%
All causes of death	247852	265917	941	692	5965	2467	17419	11505	100033	67962	123494	183291

1 May not add up to 100 due to rounding.　　* MN = malignant neoplasm.

† Suicide and undetermined injury = (E950-E959) and (E980-E989), excluding E988.8

Source: OPCS/ONS

236

Table A.2B: Five main causes of death for males and females at different ages (and percentages¹ of all causes of deaths), England, 1995

Rank	All ages – 1 and over		1-14 years		15-34 years		35-54 years		55-74 years		75 years and over	
	Males	Females	Males	Females	Males	Females	Males	Females	Males	Females	Males	Females
1	410-414 Ischaemic heart disease	410-414 Ischaemic heart disease	E800-E999 External causes of injury and poisoning	E800-999 External causes of injury and poisoning	E950-E959 Suicide and undetermined injury†	E950-959 Suicide and undetermined injury†	410-414 Ischaemic heart disease	174 MN* of female breast	410-414 Ischaemic heart disease	410-414 Ischaemic heart disease	410-414 Ischaemic heart disease	410-414 Ischaemic heart disease
	27%	21%	32%	22%	22%	11%	24%	19%	31%	21%	25%	22%
2	430-438 Cerebro-vascular disease	430-438 Cerebro-vascular disease	140-239 Neoplasms	140-239 Neoplasms	E810-E819 Motor vehicle traffic accidents	E810-E819 Motor vehicle traffic accidents	150-159 MN* of digestive organs and peritoneum	179-189 MN* of genito-urinary organs	162 MN* of trachea, bronchus and lung	150-159 MN* of digestive organs and peritoneum	480-486 Pneumonia	430-438 Cerebro-vascular disease
	8%	13%	18%	18%	16%	10%	8%	9%	11%	9%	12%	15%
3	480-486 Pneumonia	480-486 Pneumonia	320-389 Diseases of the nervous system and sense organs	740-759 Congenital anomalies	E850-E869 Accidental poisoning by drugs, medicaments and biologicals	200-208 MN* of lymphatic and haematopoietic tissue	E950-E959 Suicide and undetermined injury†	150-159 MN* of digestive organs and peritoneum	150-159 MN* of digestive organs and peritoneum	430-438 Cerebro-vascular disease	430-438 Cerebro-vascular disease	480-486 Pneumonia
	8%	11%	11%	13%	6%	5%	8%	7%	10%	8%	10%	15%
4	150-159 MN* of digestive organs and peritoneum	150-159 MN* of digestive organs and peritoneum	740-759 Congenital anomalies	320-389 Diseases of the nervous system and sense organs	001-139 Infectious and parasitic diseases	174 MN* of female breast	162 MN* of trachea, bronchus and lung	410-414 Ischaemic heart disease	430-438 Cerebro-vascular disease	162 MN* of trachea, bronchus and lung	490-496 Chronic obstructive pulmonary disease and allied conditions	415-429 Diseases of pulmonary circulation and other forms of heart disease
	8%	6%	9%	11%	5%	5%	6%	7%	6%	8%	7%	6%
5	162 MN* of trachea, bronchus and lung	415-429 Diseases of pulmonary circulation and other forms of heart disease	001-139 Infectious and parasitic diseases	460-519 Diseases of the respiratory system	200-208 MN* of lymphatic and haematopoietic tissue	179-189 MN* of genito-urinary organs	430-438 Cerebro-vascular disease	162 MN* of trachea, bronchus and lung	490-496 Chronic obstructive pulmonary disease and allied conditions	174 MN* of female breast	150-159 MN* of digestive organs and peritoneum	150-159 MN* of digestive organs and peritoneum
	8%	6%	8%	9%	4%	5%	5%	6%	6%	7%	6%	5%
Remainder	42%	43%	21%	26%	47%	63%	49%	51%	36%	46%	39%	37%
All causes of death	252458	272863	918	703	6041	2549	17935	11774	98015	66551	129549	191286

1 May not add up to 100 due to rounding.   * MN = malignant neoplasm.

† Suicide and undetermined injury = (E950-E959) and (E980-E989), excluding E988.8

Source: OPCS/ONS

Table A.3A: Relative mortality from various conditions when presented as numbers of deaths and future years of 'working life' lost, England and Wales, 1994

Cause (ICD9 code)	Males Number of deaths (thousands) All ages	(%)	Years of 'working life' lost (thousands) Age 15-64	(%)	Females Number of deaths (thousands) All ages	(%)	Years of 'working life' lost (thousands) Age 15-64	(%)
All causes, all ages	268				286			
All causes, 28 days and over	266	(100)	806	(100)	284	(100)	469	(100)
All malignant neoplasms * (140-208)	73	(27)	178	(22)	67	(24)	188	(40)
Trachea, bronchus and lung cancer (162)	21	(8)	37	(5)	11	(4)	20	(4)
Breast cancer † (174)	0	(0)	0	(0)	13	(5)	58	(12)
Genito-urinary cancer (179-189)	14	(5)	22	(3)	10	(3)	46	(10)
Leukaemia (204-208)	2	(1)	13	(2)	2	(1)	8	(2)
Circulatory disease * (390-459)	116	(44)	188	(23)	126	(44)	75	(16)
Ischaemic heart disease (410-414)	74	(28)	125	(16)	62	(22)	29	(6)
Cerebrovascular disease (430-438)	22	(8)	27	(3)	37	(13)	22	(5)
Respiratory disease * (460-519)	38	(14)	45	(6)	44	(15)	28	(6)
Pneumonia (480-486)	19	(7)	23	(3)	30	(11)	12	(3)
Bronchitis, emphysema and asthma (490-493)	4	(1)	8	(1)	3	(1)	6	(1)
Sudden infant death syndrome (798.0)	0	(0)	12	(1)	0	(0)	7	(1)
All accidental deaths * (E800-E949)	6	(2)	117	(15)	4	(2)	36	(8)
Motor vehicle traffic accidents (E810-E819)	2	(1)	60	(8)	1	(0)	20	(4)
Suicide and undetermined injury (E950-E959 plus E980-E989, excluding E988.8)	4	(1)	89	(11)	1	(0)	21	(5)

* These conditions are ranked as well as selected causes within these broader headings.   † Not calculated for male breast cancer.

Deaths under 28 days are excluded, except from 'All causes, all ages'. Method of calculation changed to that set out in DH1 (Mortality Statistics: General: England and Wales).

Source: OPCS/ONS

Table A.3B: Relative mortality from various conditions when presented as numbers of deaths and future years of 'working life' lost, England and Wales, 1995

Cause (ICD9 code)	Males				Females			
	Number of deaths (thousands)		Years of 'working life' lost (thousands)		Number of deaths (thousands)		Years of 'working life' lost (thousands)	
	All ages	(%)	Age 15-64	(%)	All ages	(%)	Age 15-64	(%)
All causes, all ages	273		892		293		531	
All causes, 28 days and over	271	(100)	815	(100)	292	(100)	473	(100)
All malignant neoplasms * (140-208)	72	(27)	171	(21)	66	(23)	188	(40)
Trachea, bronchus and lung cancer (162)	20	(8)	35	(4)	11	(4)	19	(4)
Breast cancer† (174)	0	(0)	0	(0)	13	(4)	57	(12)
Genito-urinary cancer (179-189)	14	(5)	14	(2)	10	(3)	34	(7)
Leukaemia (204-208)	2	(1)	13	(2)	2	(1)	9	(2)
Circulatory disease * (390-459)	116	(43)	189	(23)	126	(43)	74	(16)
Ischaemic heart disease (410-414)	73	(27)	123	(15)	60	(21)	28	(6)
Cerebrovascular disease (430-438)	22	(8)	27	(3)	38	(13)	23	(5)
Respiratory disease * (460-519)	41	(15)	45	(6)	49	(17)	30	(6)
Pneumonia (480-486)	21	(8)	24	(3)	33	(11)	14	(3)
Bronchitis, emphysema and asthma (490-493)	4	(1)	6	(1)	3	(1)	6	(1)
Sudden infant death syndrome (798.0)	0	(0)	10	(1)	0	(0)	6	(1)
All accidental deaths * (E800-E949)	6	(2)	120	(15)	4	(1)	34	(7)
Motor vehicle traffic accidents (E810-E819)	2	(1)	60	(7)	1	(0)	18	(4)
Suicide and undetermined injury (E950-E959 plus E980-E989, excluding E988.8)	4	(1)	89	(11)	1	(0)	23	(5)

* These conditions are ranked as well as selected causes within these broader headings.   † Not calculated for male breast cancer.

Deaths under 28 days are excluded, except from 'All causes, all ages'. Method of calculation changed to that set out in DH1 (Mortality Statistics: General: England and Wales).

Source: OPCS/ONS

Table A.4: *Trends in 'avoidable' deaths, England, 1979-95. Age-standardised mortality ratios (1979 = 100)*

Condition	SMR[1]													Actual number of deaths[2]	
	1979	1984	1985	1986	1987	1988	1989	1990	1991	1992	1993	1994	1995[3]	1979	1995[4]
Hypertension/cerebrovascular (ages 35-64)	100	77	76	73	69	63	60	57	58	55	52	49	49	8811	4329
Perinatal mortality[5]	100	69	67	65	61	60	57	56	55	52	52[6]	52[6]	51[6]	8839	4555[6]
Cervical cancer (ages 15-64)	100	91	90	96	90	86	81	78	72	68	64	53	56	1060	613
Hodgkin's disease (ages 5-64)	100	81	77	75	84	74	65	60	58	57	60	39	49	340	181
Respiratory diseases (ages 1-14)	100	51	50	41	44	42	41	39	42	28	44	48	36	308	115
Surgical diseases[7] (ages 5-64)	100	78	65	71	58	75	51	58	58	61	54	45	52	247	128
Asthma (ages 5-44)	100	105	115	114	114	110	94	86	91	70	68	64	47	231	117
Tuberculosis (ages 5-64)	100	67	67	60	67	56	57	48	46	47	53	50	56	208	120
Chronic rheumatic heart disease (ages 5-44)	100	43	34	35	34	20	28	23	19	14	17	19	17	118	23
Total 'avoidable' deaths	100	74	72	70	66	63	60	57	57	54	53	50	50	20138[8]	10167[8]
All causes: ages 0-14 years	100	76	75	74	73	72	67	64	59	52	52	49	49	10502	5338
All causes: ages 15-64 years	100	88	88	86	84	82	80	79	76	74	73	70	70	119158	84424
All causes: all ages	100	89	92	89	86	85	85	82	82	79	81	77	78	554840	529038

[1] The standardised mortality ratio (SMR) for a condition is calculated by dividing the observed number of deaths by the expected number of deaths based on 1979 death rates.

[2] Excluding deaths of visitors to England.

[3] 1995 population projections (1994 based) were used to calculate the 1995 SMRs as estimates not yet available.

[4] From 1993 the mortality data for some causes of death are not directly comparable with those for 1992 and earlier years as a result of coding changes.

[5] Stillbirths are included in the figures for perinatal mortality and total 'avoidable' deaths, but not in deaths from all causes.

[6] The definition of stillbirth changed on 1 October 1992 to include 24 to 27 weeks gestation; to provide a comparable trend, these stillbirths are excluded from the figures for 1993 (848), 1994 (832) and 1995 (842).

[7] Appendicitis, abdominal hernia, cholelithiasis and cholecystitis.

[8] Figures for total 'avoidable' deaths take account of deaths from asthma in the 5-14 age band already counted in the figures for respiratory diseases.

Source: Department of Health, from data supplied by OPCS/ONS

Table A.5: Live births, stillbirths, infant mortality and abortions, England[1], 1960, 1970, 1975–95

Year	Live births Number	Stillbirths Number	Stillbirths Rate[2]	Early neonatal mortality (deaths under 1 week) Number	Early neonatal mortality (deaths under 1 week) Rate[3]	Perinatal mortality (stillbirths plus deaths under 1 week) Rate[2]	Post-neonatal mortality (deaths 4 weeks to under 1 year) Rate[3]	Infant mortality (deaths under 1 year) Rate[3]	Abortions[1] Rate[4]
1960	740859	14753	19.5	9772	13.2	32.5	6.3	21.6	-
1970	741999	9708	12.9	7864	10.6	23.4	5.9	18.2	87.6
1975	563900	5918	10.4	5154	9.1	19.4	5.0	15.7	149.9
1976	550393	5339	9.6	4468	8.1	17.6	4.6	14.2	148.7
1977	536953	5087	9.4	4070	7.6	16.9	4.5	13.7	152.7
1978	562589	4791	8.4	3975	7.1	15.4	4.4	13.1	157.7
1979	601316	4811	7.9	4028	6.7	14.6	4.5	12.8	158.8
1980	619371	4523	7.3	3793	6.1	13.4	4.4	12.0	164.5
1981	598163	3939	6.5	3105	5.2	11.7	4.3	10.9	168.8
1982	589711	3731	6.3	2939	5.0	11.2	4.5*	10.8	171.1
1983	593255	3412	5.7	2746	4.6	10.3	4.2	10.0	169.2
1984	600573	3425	5.7	2640	4.4	10.0	3.9	9.4	177.3
1985	619301	3426	5.5	2674	4.3	9.8	3.9	9.2	177.6
1986	623609	3337	5.3	2640	4.2	9.5	4.2	9.5	183.5
1987	643330	3224	5.0	2518	3.9	8.9	4.0	9.1	187.7
1988	654360	3188	4.8	2543	3.9	8.7	4.1	9.1	196.6
1989	649357	3056	4.7	2368	3.6	8.3	3.7	8.4	200.0
1990	666920	3068	4.6	2382	3.6	8.1	3.3	7.9	199.0
1991	660806	3072	4.6	2260	3.4	8.0	3.0	7.3	194.4
1992	651784†	2777†	4.2†	2174	3.3	7.6†	2.3	6.5	190.1
1993[5]	636614	3632	5.7	2075	3.3	8.9	2.1	6.3	190.8
1994[5]	628693	3584	5.7	2014	3.2	8.9	2.0	6.1	193.8
1995[6]	613239	3406	5.5	1996	3.3	8.8	1.9	6.1	-

[1] Relates to England residents.   [2] Per 1,000 live births and stillbirths.   [3] Per 1,000 live births.   [4] Per 1,000 conceptions (live births, stillbirths and abortions).

[5] 1993 and 1994 figures are slightly different from those published in the previous Report as they are derived from a live database.   [6] Provisional.

* The post-neonatal mortality rate in 1982 has been incorrectly cited as 4.6 per 1,000 live births in recent Reports.

† 1992 figures exclude 198 stillbirths of between 24 and 27 completed weeks gestation registered between 1 October 1992 and 31 December 1992, following the introduction of new legislation (see Chapter 1), and are consistent with those for earlier years. The figures for later years are on the new (wider) definition of stillbirths.

Source: OPCS/ONS

241

Table A.6: *Congenital anomalies, England, 1985, 1990, 1994* and 1995**

ICD code(s)	Anomaly	Live births†				Stillbirths§			
		1985	1990	1994	1995¶	1985	1990	1994	1995¶
	Babies born with anomalies								
	Number	12215	7518	5114	4950	322	199	179	165
	Rate	197.2	112.7	81.3	80.7	5.2	3.0	2.8	2.7
320.0-359.9, 740.0-742.9 (Q00.0 - Q07.9)	**Central nervous system**								
	Number	549	266	181	169	114	54	44	48
	Rate	8.9	4.0	2.9	2.8	1.8	0.8	0.7	0.8
360.0-379.9, 743.0-743.9, 744.0-744.3 (Q10.0 - Q17.9)	**Ear and eye**								
	Number	669	382	210	187	16	11	6	9
	Rate	10.8	5.7	3.3	3.0	0.3	0.2	0.1	0.1
749.0-749.2 (Q35.0 - Q37.9)	**Cleft lip/cleft palate**								
	Number	741	691	567	524	18	17	20	6
	Rate	12.0	10.4	9.0	8.5	0.3	0.3	0.3	0.1
390.0-459.9, 745.0-747.9 (Q20.0 - Q28.9)	**Cardiovascular**								
	Number	649	454	371	380	12	20	20	13
	Rate	10.5	6.8	5.9	6.2	0.2	0.3	0.3	0.2
752.6 (Q54.0 - Q54.9, Q64.0)	**Hypospadias/epispadias**								
	Number	1001	818	516	461	3	1	1	0
	Rate	16.2	12.3	8.2	7.5	0.0	0.0	0.0	-
755.2-755.4 (Q71.0 - Q73.8)	**Reduction deformities of limbs**								
	Number	299	180	178	175	7	3	6	5
	Rate	4.8	2.7	2.8	2.9	0.1	0.0	0.1	0.1
754.5-754.7 (Q66.0, Q66.1, Q66.4, Q66.8)	**Talipes**								
	Number	1873	992	677	641	19	10	9	5
	Rate	30.2	14.9	10.8	10.5	0.3	0.1	0.1	0.1
758.0-758.9 (Q90.0 - Q99.9)	**Chromosomal**								
	Number	520	470	365	359	15	21	26	27
	Rate	8.4	7.0	5.8	5.9	0.2	0.3	0.4	0.4

* From January 1990 certain minor malformations are no longer notified, and have been excluded from the figures shown. For example, club foot of positional origin is now excluded from the category 'Talipes', ICD Codes 754.5-754.7. This change in notification practice largely accounts for the decrease in the number of malformations reported in some categories. From 1995 ICD 10 codes (in brackets) are in use.

† Rates per 10,000 live births. § Rates per 10,000 total births. ¶ Provisional data.

Source: OPCS/ONS

Table A.7: Cancer* registrations by age and site, males, England and Wales, 1991

Numbers and percentages

	All ages	%	0-14 years	%	15-24 years	%	25-44 years	%	45-64 years	%	65-74 years	%	75-84 years	%	85 years and over	%
Eye, brain and other nervous system	2115	2	142	21	80	10	320	7	824	3	496	1	230	1	23	0
Mouth and pharynx	2146	2	5	1	15	2	129	3	923	4	603	2	406	2	65	1
Oesophagus	3134	3	0	0	0	0	68	2	872	3	1160	3	821	3	213	3
Lung	24751	24	2	0	4	1	328	7	6195	24	9500	27	7277	24	1445	20
Stomach	6138	6	0	0	2	0	103	2	1493	6	2068	6	1981	7	491	7
Pancreas	3051	3	1	0	1	0	61	1	799	3	1071	3	912	3	206	3
Large intestine and rectum	13895	13	1	0	6	1	375	8	3733	14	4772	14	4034	13	974	13
Prostate	13940	13	3	0	2	0	11	0	1590	6	4816	14	5835	20	1683	23
Bladder	8289	8	2	0	6	1	162	4	2044	8	2896	8	2517	8	662	9
Skin (melanoma)†	1468	1	3	0	41	5	316	7	562	2	295	1	195	1	56	1
Leukaemias and lymphomas	8509	8	318	47	307	39	924	21	2246	9	2216	6	1964	7	534	7
All other cancer	16774	16	196	29	319	41	1685	38	4716	18	5118	15	3738	12	1002	14
Total cancer	104210	100	673	100	783	100	4482	100	25997	100	35011	100	29910	100	7354	100

* Cancer = malignant neoplasm.

† Melanoma of skin only (ICD9 code 172). Earlier Reports included figures for other malignant neoplasm of skin (ICD9 code 173), which are greatly under-registered.

Note: Percentages may not add up to 100 due to rounding.

Source: OPCS/ONS

243

Table A.8: *Cancer* registrations by age and site, females, England and Wales, 1991*

Numbers and percentages

	Age-group (years)															
	All ages	%	0-14 years	%	15-24 years	%	25-44 years	%	45-64 years	%	65-74 years	%	75-84 years	%	85 years and over	%
Eye, brain and other nervous system	1636	2	139	26	60	9	250	3	576	2	361	1	209	1	41	0
Mouth and pharynx	1185	2	7	1	5	1	87	1	341	1	303	1	299	1	143	1
Oesophagus	2226	2	0	0	0	0	23	0	378	1	583	2	839	3	403	4
Breast	30595	28	1	0	27	4	3470	41	13512	42	6328	23	5021	19	2236	19
Lung	11754	11	0	0	7	1	173	2	2961	9	4438	16	3323	12	852	7
Stomach	3924	4	0	0	1	0	82	1	540	2	965	3	1474	6	862	8
Pancreas	3216	3	1	0	2	0	45	1	590	2	918	3	1132	4	528	5
Large intestine and rectum	13844	13	1	0	10	1	325	4	2769	9	3841	14	4631	17	2267	20
Ovary	5277	5	3	1	44	7	450	5	2089	6	1373	5	1013	4	305	3
Cervix	3768	3	0	0	49	7	1403	17	1147	4	651	2	416	2	102	1
Other uterus	4282	4	1	0	8	1	167	2	1668	5	1241	4	882	3	315	3
Bladder	3180	3	0	0	6	1	61	1	597	2	945	3	1088	4	483	4
Skin (melanoma)†	2235	2	7	1	82	12	598	7	685	2	395	2	344	1	124	1
Leukaemias and lymphomas	7013	7	208	39	231	34	577	7	1520	5	1745	6	1950	7	782	7
All other cancer	13724	13	172	32	139	21	764	9	2803	9	3656	13	4149	15	2041	18
Total cancer	107859	100	540	100	671	100	8475	100	32176	100	27743	100	26770	100	11484	100

* Cancer = malignant neoplasm.

† Melanoma of skin only (ICD9 code 172). Earlier Reports included figures for other malignant neoplasm of skin (ICD9 code 173), which are greatly under-registered.

Note: Percentages may not add up to 100 due to rounding.

Source: OPCS/ONS

Table A.9: *Percentage of children immunised by their 2nd birthday and of children given BCG vaccine by their 14th birthday, England, 1980-94/95*

Year	Diphtheria	Tetanus	Polio	Whooping cough	Measles	Mumps/rubella	BCG[1]
1980[2]	81	81	81	41	53	-	82
1981[2]	83	83	82	46	55	-	78
1982[2]	84	84	84	53	58	-	75
1983[2]	84	84	84	59	60	-	76
1984[2]	84	84	84	65	63	-	71
1985[2]	85	85	85	65	68	-	77
1986[2]	85	85	85	67	71	-	76
1987/88[2]	87	87	87	73	76	-	76
1988/89	87	87	87	75	80	7	71
1989/90	89	89	89	78	84	68	36[3]
1990/91	92	92	92	84	87	86	90[3]
1991/92	93	93	93	88	90	90	86[3]
1992/93	95	95	95	92	92	92	74
1993/94	95	95	95	93	91	91	79
1994/95	95	95	95	93	91	91	52[4]

[1] Estimated percentage.

[2] Estimated percentage immunised by the end of the second year after birth.

[3] The school BCG programme was suspended in 1989 because there were insufficient supplies of BCG vaccine; figures for the subsequent two years were relatively higher as a result.

[4] The school BCG programme for 1994/95 was delayed as a result of the measles/rubella immunisation campaign.

Sources: 1980-87/88: Form SBL 607

1988/89 onwards: Form KC51 (except BCG); KC50 (BCG)

Table A.10: *Cumulative totals of AIDS cases by exposure category, England, to 31 December 1995*

(Numbers subject to revision as further data are received or duplicates identified)

How persons probably acquired the virus	Number of cases			
	Male	Female	Total	%§
Sexual intercourse:				
Between men	7995	-	7995	73
Between men and women				
Exposure to				
'high risk' partner*	34	107	141	1
Exposure abroad†	661	487	1148	11
Exposure in the UK	65	55	120	1
Investigation continuing/closed	21	4	25	<1
Injecting drug use (IDU)	303	131	434	4
IDU and sexual intercourse				
between men	182	-	182	2
Blood factor treatment				
(eg for haemophilia)	487	5	492	5
Blood/tissue transfer				
(eg transfusion)				
Abroad	14	41	55	<1
UK	21	23	44	<1
Mother to infant	83	85	168	2
Other or investigation continuing/				
closed	92	19	111	1
Total	9958	957	10915	100

* Partner(s) exposed to HIV infection through sexual intercourse between men, IDU, blood factor treatment or blood/tissue transfer.

† Individuals from abroad and individuals from the UK who have lived or visited abroad, for whom there is no evidence of 'high risk' partners.

§ Total does not add up to 100 because of rounding.

Source: CDSC/PHLS

Table A.11: *Expectation of life at birth, all-cause death rates and infant mortality, England and other European Union countries, circa 1993*

Country	Year	Expection of life at birth		All cause mortality rate*		Infant mortality rate**
		Males	Females	Males	Females	
England	1994	74.5†	79.7†	281.8§	171.6§	6.1§
United Kingdom	1992	73.6	79.2	311.6	186.7	6.6
Austria	1994	73.4	79.9	349.4	165.3	6.3
Belgium	1989	72.3	79.1	353.4	184.2	8.5
Denmark	1993	72.7	77.9	351.9	228.8	5.4
Finland	1993	72.1	79.6	385.1	155.7	4.4
France	1992	73.8	82.3	370.9	150.4	6.8
Germany	1994	73.1	79.7	356.0	169.8	5.1
Greece	1993	75.0	80.4	289.0	135.8	8.3
Ireland	1992	72.6	78.2	325.8	192.0	6.7
Italy	1991	73.7	80.5	327.0	151.8	8.2
Luxembourg	1993	72.4	79.3	357.4	181.3	5.2
Netherlands	1993	74.0	80.1	288.1	165.5	6.3
Portugal	1993	70.6	77.9	432.0	192.7	8.7
Spain	1992	73.8	81.3	342.8	138.6	7.1
Sweden	1992	75.5	81.1	262.5	149.1	5.2
EU average	*1993*	*73.4*	*80.2*	*342.9*	*164.8*	*6.8*

* Per 100,000 population aged 0-64 years, age-standardised.

**Per 1,000 live births.

† Figure for England calculated by Government Actuary's Department by slightly different methodology to WHO figures.

§ England data provided by OPCS/ONS.

Source: WHO European Office 'Health for All' statistical database

247

Figure A1: *Weekly deaths, England and Wales, 1994 and 1995, and expected deaths, 1995*

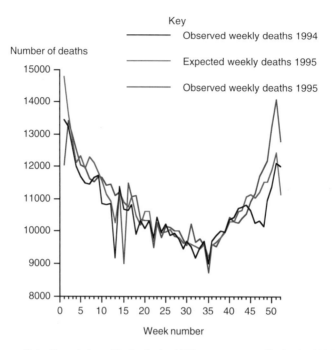

Note: Expected weekly deaths for 1995 = average weekly deaths 1990-94

Source: OPCS/ONS

Printed in the UK for HMSO
Dd 302970 C30 9/96 3400/3 13110